Medical Surgical Nursing

Practical Record Book

for BSc/Diploma Nursing Students

Siddusing S Hajeri MSc Nursing (Medical Surgical Nursing)

Professor and Head
Department of Medical Surgical Nursing and Principal
Shri JG Co-operative Hospital Society's College of Nursing
Ghataprabha, Belgaum, Karnataka

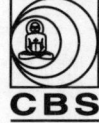

CBS Publishers & Distributors Pvt Ltd

New Delhi • Bengaluru • Chennai • Kochi • Kolkata • Mumbai
Hyderabad • Nagpur • Patna • Pune • Vijayawada

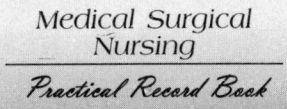

Medical Surgical Nursing
Practical Record Book

ISBN: 978-81-239-2957-6

First Edition: 2016

Published by Satish Kumar Jain and Produced by Varun Jain for

CBS Publishers & Distributors Pvt Ltd

4819/XI Prahlad Street, 24 Ansari Road, Daryaganj, New Delhi 110 002, India.

Ph: 23289259, 23266861, 23266867   Fax: 011-23243014   Website: www.cbspd.com
e-mail: delhi@cbspd.com; cbspubs@airtelmail.in.

Corporate Office: 204 FIE, Industrial Area, Patparganj, Delhi 110 092

Ph: 4934 4934   Fax: 4934 4935   e-mail: publishing@cbspd.com;   publicity@cbspd.com

Branches

• **Bengaluru:** Seema House 2975, 17th Cross, K.R. Road, Banasankari 2nd Stage, Bengaluru 560 070, Karnataka
Ph: +91-80-26771678/79   Fax: +91-80-26771680   e-mail: bangalore@cbspd.com

• **Chennai:** No. 7, Subbaraya Street, Shenoy Nagar, Chennai 600 030, Tamil Nadu
Ph: +91-44-26680620, 26681266   Fax: +91-44-42032115   e-mail: chennai@cbspd.com

• **Kochi:** Ashana House, 39/1904, AM Thomas Road, Valanjambalam, Ernakulam 682 018, Kochi, Kerala
Ph: +91-484-4059061-62-64-65   Fax: +91-484-4059065   e-mail: kochi@cbspd.com

• **Kolkata:** No. 6/B, Ground Floor, Rameswar Shaw Road, Kolkata-700014 (West Bengal), India
Ph: +91-33-2289-1126, 2289-1127, 2289-1128   e-mail: kolkata@cbspd.com

• **Mumbai:** 83-C, Dr E Moses Road, Worli, Mumbai-400018, Maharashtra
Ph: +91-22-24902340/41   Fax: +91-22-24902342   e-mail: mumbai@cbspd.com

Representatives

• **Hyderabad**   0-9885175004   • **Nagpur**   0-9021734563   • **Patna**   0-9334159340
• **Pune**   0-9623451994   • **Vijayawada**   0-9000660880

Printed at : Swastik Packagings, 506 F.I.E., Patparganj, Delhi - 110092

Student Profile

Photograph

Name of the college	:	....
		....
Name of the student	:	....
Registration No.	:	....
Age and date of birth	:	....
Religion	:	....
Father's name	:	....
Mother's name	:	....
Mother tongue	:	....
Date of joining course	:	....
Date of stating clinical posting	:	....
Date of completion of clinical posting	:	....
Permanent address	:	....

Signature of the Student	**Signature of the Teacher**
Signature of the HOD	**Signature of the Principal**
Signature of the Internal Examiner	**Signature of the External Examiner**

Preface

It gives me immense pleasure and satisfaction to introduce the *Medical Surgical Nursing Practical Record Book* for BSc Nursing/Diploma Nursing Students which will enable the student to meet the clinical requirement for partial fulfilment of their requirement in the medical surgical nursing subject.

Nursing is an applied science, knowledge which is acquired in the classroom to be put into practice in their clinical setup while in their respective clinical posting, hence there is a need of objectives for clinical experiences in the hospital or health care setup.

My aim for preparing this clinical record book to acquaint all nursing students with knowledge and skills in providing nursing care to the assigned clients and who comes their clinical settings.

This book can be used for clinical records of their experiences during the clinical postings in the medical surgical nursing, which will help the students to write their prescribed assignments.

I have tried my best to provide the basic instruments and guidelines to prepare their assignment in a proper way in the annexures.

I hope this book will be beneficial to the students in their selected nursing courses.

Siddusing S Hajeri

Clinical Objectives

1.	• Provide nursing care to adult patients with medical disorders • Counsel and educate patients and families
2.	• Provide pre- and postoperative nursing care to adult patients with surgical disorders • Counsel and educate patients and families
3.	• Provide nursing care to patients with cardiac disorders • Counsel and educate patients and families
4.	• Identify skin problems • Provide nursing care to patients with skin disorders and communicable diseases • Counsel and educate patients and families
5.	• Provide nursing care to patients with musculoskeletal disorders • Counsel and educate patients and families
6.	• Identify instruments used in common operations • Participate in infection control practices in the operation theatre • Setup the table/trolleys for common operative procedures • Assist in giving anesthesia • Assist in the operative procedures • Provide perioperative nursing care
7.	• To gain proficiency in ICU nursing • Develop advance skill in special procedures used in critical care unit • Identify potential problems and provide accordingly • Skill in setting and handling ventilator • Administer injection in infusion pump • Record accurately findings and medications • Develop IPR with family members • Acquaint with OT technique
8.	• Develop skill in neurological assessment • Give care to the patient with head injury and spinal injury • Care with chest surgery and cranial surgery
9.	• Assess the severity of burns • Administer rehydration therapy • Observe reconstructive surgery
10.	• Identify instruments • Assist in OT set up • Supervise sterilization • Assist in OT table layout • Observe immediately after operation • Supervise infection control
11.	• Provide care to patients with ENT disorders • Counsel and educate patient and families
12.	• Provide care to patients with eye disorders • Counsel and educate patient and families

13.	• Provide care to patients with neurological disorders • Counsel and educate patient and families
14.	• Provide care to patients with gynecological disorders • Counsel and educate patient and families
15.	• Provide care to patients with burns • Counsel and educate patient and families
16.	• Provide care to patients with cancer • Counsel and educate patient and families
17.	• Provide care to critically ill patients • Counsel patient and families for grief and bereavement
18.	• Provide care to patients in emergency and disaster situation • Counsel patient and families for grief and bereavement

Contents

Nursing Care Plan 1

I. Identification data:

a. Name : ....

b. Address : ....

c. Age : ....

d. Sex : ....

e. Marital status : ....

f. Education : ....

g. Occupation : ....

h. Income : ....

i. Religion : ....

j. IP No. : ....

k. Diagnosis : ....

l. Date of admission : ....

II. Presenting chief complaints: [Write down the client's problem as per their verbatim in chronological order.]

_____

_____

_____

III. History of present illness: Explain the client's problem with aggravating factors, relieving factor, precipitating factors, its characteristics, intensity, etc.

_____

_____

_____

_____

_____

IV. **Past history of illness:** Explain the past medical, surgical history with its treatment, etc.

_____

_____

_____

_____

_____

_____

_____

V. **Family history:** [Family structure/family health history/social support system, etc.]

Index	
⊘	Client
○	Female
□	Male

Sl. No.	Name of the family members	Relationship with patient	Age/sex	Educational status	Occupational status	Marital status	Health status
1.							
2.							
3.							
4.							
5.							
6.							
7.							
8.							
9.							
10.							

VI. **Personal history:** [Bowel, bladder, sleep, diet, habit, etc.]

_____

_____

_____

_____

_____

_____

PHYSICAL EXAMINATION

General Appearance

Level of consciousness : ....

Activity : ....

Body built : ....

Height : ....

Weight : ....

General grooming : ....

Body language : ....

Other observations : ....

Skin

Colour and vascularity : ....

Turgor and mobility : ....

Temperature and moisture : ....

Texture : ....

Nails : ....

Body hair growth : ....

Skin integrity : ....

Lesions : ....

Head

Shape : ....

Face : ....

Sensation : ....

Hair : ....

Condition of the scalp : ....

Facial puffiness : ....

Eyes

Eyebrows : ....

Eyelashes : ....

Eyelids : ....

Shape and appearance : ....

Sclera : ....

conjunctiva : ....

Iris : ....

Cornea : ....

Pupils : ....

Visual field : ....

Vision : ....

Use of glasses : ....

Ears

Pinnae : ....

Level in relation to eyes : ....

Canal : ....

Cilia : ....

Cerumen : ....

Tympanic membrane : ....

Hearing (audition) : ....

Tuning fork test : ....

Weber test : ....

Rinne test : ....

Hearing aid : ....

Nose and Sinuses

Size and shape : ....

Nasal septum : ....

Nasal mucosa and turbinate : ....

Patency of nares : ....

Olfactory : ....

Sinuses : ....

Mouth and Pharynx

Lips : ....

Teeth : ....

Dental caries and fillings : ....

Dental hygiene : ....

Breath odor : ....

Gums : ....

Facial and glossopharyngeal
nerve : ....

Tongue : ....

Hypoglossal : ....

Mucosa : ....

Palate : ....

Uvula : ....

Pharynx : ....

Tonsils : ....

Temporomandibular joint : ....

Neck

Appearance : ....

Thyroid : ....

Trachea : ....

Lymph nodes : ....

Thorax and Lungs

Respiratory rate : ....

Thoracic cage shape : ....

Configuration : ....

Skin color and condition : ....

Chest examination : ....

Posterior thorax : ....

Percussion of lung field : ....

Diaphragmatic exertion : ....

Lung auscultation : ....

Breath sound : ....

Respiratory pattern

Breast and Axillae

Male breasts : ....

Female breasts : ....

Nipples : ....

Axillae : ....

Cardiovascular Examination

Heart : ....

Heart sound : ....

Murmurs : ....

Carotid pulse : ....

Apical pulse : ....

Peripheral pulses : ....

Blood pressure : ....

Abdominal Examinations

Contour : ....

Skin : ....

Bowel sounds : ....

On percussion : ....

Palpation : ....

Musculoskeletal Examination

Back : ....

Vertebral column alignment : ....

Range of motion : ....

Extremities : ....

Lower extremities : ....

Genitourinary and Rectum

Rectum : ....

Female genitalia : ....

Male genitalia : ....

Neurological Examination

Describes tics, twitches, paresthesias : ....

Gait : ....

Cranial nerves : ....

Reflexes : ....

Co-ordination : ....

Mental Status Examination

Level of alertness : ....

Orientation : ....

Memory : ....

Language and speech : ....

Responsiveness : ....

Knowledge test   : ....

Thinking   : ....

Judgment   : ....

Insight   : ....

Investigation

Sl. No.	Name of investigation	Client's value	Normal value	Remarks
1.				
2.				
3.				
4.				
5.				
6.				
7.				
8.				
9.				
10.				

Treatment/Medications

Sl. No.	Name of drug	Dosage	Frequency	Class of drug
1.				
2.				
3.				
4.				
5.				
6.				
7.				
8.				
9.				
10.				

Nursing diagnosis: List down the nursing diagnosis based on needs and problems of the client with priority [Maslow's hierarchy].

Care plan: Prepare the plan of care with priority [at least 5 need-based care to be given].

Assessment	Diagnosis	Objectives	Intervention	Rationale	Evaluation

Assessment	Diagnosis	Objectives	Intervention	Rationale	Evaluation

Health Education: List down the health education topics, prepare AV aids and impart the education.

Nursing Care Plan 2

I. Identification data:

    a. Name   : ....

    b. Address   : ....

    c. Age   : ....

    d. Sex   : ....

    e. Marital status : ....

    f. Education   : ....

    g. Occupation   : ....

    h. Income   : ....

    i. Religion   : ....

    j. IP No.   : ....

    k. Diagnosis   : ....

    l. Date of admission : ....

II. Presenting chief complaints: [Write down the client's problem as per their verbatim in chronological order.]

_____

_____

_____

III. History of present illness: Explain the client's problem with aggravating factors, relieving factor, precipitating factors, its characteristics, intensity, etc.

_____

_____

_____

_____

_____

_____

IV. **Past history of illness:** Explain the past medical, surgical history with its treatment, etc.

_____

_____

_____

_____

_____

_____

_____

V. **Family history:** [Family structure/family health history/social support system, etc.]

Index	
⊘	Client
◯	Female
☐	Male

Sl. No.	Name of the family members	Relationship with patient	Age/sex	Educational status	Occupational status	Marital status	Health status
1.							
2.							
3.							
4.							
5.							
6.							
7.							
8.							
9.							
10.							

VI. **Personal history:** [Bowel, bladder, sleep, diet, habit, etc.]

_____

_____

_____

_____

_____

_____

_____

PHYSICAL EXAMINATION

General Appearance

Level of consciousness   : ....

Activity   : ....

Body built   : ....

Height   : ....

Weight   : ....

General grooming   : ....

Body language   : ....

Other observations   : ....

Skin

Colour and vascularity   : ....

Turgor and mobility   : ....

Temperature and moisture   : ....

Texture   : ....

Nails   : ....

Body hair growth   : ....

Skin integrity   : ....

Lesions   : ....

Head

Shape   : ....

Face   : ....

Sensation   : ....

Hair   : ....

Condition of the scalp   : ....

Facial puffiness   : ....

Eyes

Eyebrows   : ....

Eyelashes   : ....

Eyelids   : ....

Shape and appearance   : ....

Sclera   : ....

conjunctiva   : ....

Iris   : ....

Cornea   : ....

Pupils   : ....

Visual field   : ....

Vision   : ....

Use of glasses   : ....

Ears

Pinnae   : ....

Level in relation to eyes   : ....

Canal   : ....

Cilia   : ....

Cerumen   : ....

Tympanic membrane   : ....

Hearing (audition)   : ....

Tuning fork test   : ....

Weber test   : ....

Rinne test   : ....

Hearing aid   : ....

Nose and Sinuses

Size and shape   : ....

Nasal septum   : ....

Nasal mucosa and turbinate   : ....

Patency of nares   : ....

Olfactory   : ....

Sinuses   : ....

Mouth and Pharynx

Lips   : ....

Teeth   : ....

Dental caries and fillings   : ....

Dental hygiene   : ....

Breath odor   : ....

Gums   : ....

Facial and glossopharyngeal
nerve   : ....

Tongue   : ....

Hypoglossal   : ....

Mucosa   : ....

Palate   : ....

Uvula : ....

Pharynx : ....

Tonsils : ....

Temporomandibular joint : ....

Neck

Appearance : ....

Thyroid : ....

Trachea : ....

Lymph nodes : ....

Thorax and Lungs

Respiratory rate : ....

Thoracic cage shape : ....

Configuration : ....

Skin color and condition : ....

Chest examination : ....

Posterior thorax : ....

Percussion of lung field : ....

Diaphragmatic exertion : ....

Lung auscultation : ....

Breath sound : ....

Respiratory pattern

Breast and Axillae

Male breasts : ....

Female breasts : ....

Nipples : ....

Axillae : ....

Cardiovascular Examination

Heart : ....

Heart sound : ....

Murmurs : ....

Carotid pulse : ....

Apical pulse : ....

Peripheral pulses : ....

Blood pressure : ....

Abdominal Examinations

Contour   : ....

Skin   : ....

Bowel sounds   : ....

On percussion   : ....

Palpation   : ....

Musculoskeletal Examination

Back   : ....

Vertebral column alignment   : ....

Range of motion   : ....

Extremities   : ....

Lower extremities   : ....

Genitourinary and Rectum

Rectum   : ....

Female genitalia   : ....

Male genitalia   : ....

Neurological Examination

Describes tics,
twitches, paresthesias   : ....

Gait   : ....

Cranial nerves   : ....

Reflexes   : ....

Co-ordination   : ....

Mental Status Examination

Level of alertness   : ....

Orientation   : ....

Memory   : ....

Language and speech   : ....

Responsiveness   : ....

Knowledge test   : ....

Thinking   : ....

Judgment   : ....

Insight   : ....

Investigation

Sl. No.	Name of investigation	Client's value	Normal value	Remarks
1.				
2.				
3.				
4.				
5.				
6.				
7.				
8.				
9.				
10.				

Treatment/Medications

Sl. No.	Name of drug	Dosage	Frequency	Class of drug
1.				
2.				
3.				
4.				
5.				
6.				
7.				
8.				
9.				
10.				

Nursing diagnosis: List down the nursing diagnosis based on needs and problems of the client with priority [Maslow's hierarchy].

Care plan: Prepare the plan of care with priority [at least 5 need-based care to be given].

Assessment	Diagnosis	Objectives	Intervention	Rationale	Evaluation

Assessment	Diagnosis	Objectives	Intervention	Rationale	Evaluation

Health Education: List down the health education topics, prepare AV aids and impart the education.

Nursing Care Plan 3

HISTORY TAKING

I. Identification data:

a. Name : ....

b. Address : ....

c. Age : ....

d. Sex : ....

e. Marital status : ....

f. Education : ....

g. Occupation : ....

h. Income : ....

i. Religion : ....

j. IP No. : ....

k. Diagnosis : ....

l. Date of admission : ....

II. Presenting chief complaints: [Write down the client's problem as per their verbatim in chronological order.]

_____

_____

_____

III. History of present illness: Explain the client's problem with aggravating factors, relieving factor, precipitating factors, its characteristics, intensity, etc.

_____

_____

_____

_____

_____

_____

IV. **Past history of illness:** Explain the past medical, surgical history with its treatment, etc.

_____

_____

_____

_____

_____

_____

_____

V. **Family history:** [Family structure/family health history/social support system, etc.]

Index	
⊘	Client
◯	Female
▢	Male

Sl. No.	Name of the family members	Relationship with patient	Age/sex	Educational status	Occupational status	Marital status	Health status
1.							
2.							
3.							
4.							
5.							
6.							
7.							
8.							
9.							
10.							

VI. **Personal history:** [Bowel, bladder, sleep, diet, habit, etc.]

_____

_____

_____

_____

_____

_____

PHYSICAL EXAMINATION

General Appearance

Level of consciousness : ....

Activity : ....

Body built : ....

Height : ....

Weight : ....

General grooming : ....

Body language : ....

Other observations : ....

Skin

Colour and vascularity : ....

Turgor and mobility : ....

Temperature and moisture : ....

Texture : ....

Nails : ....

Body hair growth : ....

Skin integrity : ....

Lesions : ....

Head

Shape : ....

Face : ....

Sensation : ....

Hair : ....

Condition of the scalp : ....

Facial puffiness : ....

Eyes

Eyebrows : ....

Eyelashes : ....

Eyelids : ....

Shape and appearance : ....

Sclera : ....

conjunctiva : ....

Iris : ....

Cornea : ....

Pupils : ....

Visual field : ....

Vision : ....

Use of glasses : ....

Ears

Pinnae : ....

Level in relation to eyes : ....

Canal : ....

Cilia : ....

Cerumen : ....

Tympanic membrane : ....

Hearing (audition) : ....

Tuning fork test : ....

Weber test : ....

Rinne test : ....

Hearing aid : ....

Nose and Sinuses

Size and shape : ....

Nasal septum : ....

Nasal mucosa and turbinate : ....

Patency of nares : ....

Olfactory : ....

Sinuses : ....

Mouth and Pharynx

Lips : ....

Teeth : ....

Dental caries and fillings : ....

Dental hygiene : ....

Breath odor : ....

Gums : ....

Facial and glossopharyngeal
nerve : ....

Tongue : ....

Hypoglossal : ....

Mucosa : ....

Palate : ....

Uvula   : ....

Pharynx   : ....

Tonsils   : ....

Temporomandibular joint   : ....

Neck

Appearance   : ....

Thyroid   : ....

Trachea   : ....

Lymph nodes   : ....

Thorax and Lungs

Respiratory rate   : ....

Thoracic cage shape   : ....

Configuration   : ....

Skin color and condition   : ....

Chest examination   : ....

Posterior thorax   : ....

Percussion of lung field   : ....

Diaphragmatic exertion   : ....

Lung auscultation   : ....

Breath sound   : ....

Respiratory pattern

Breast and Axillae

Male breasts   : ....

Female breasts   : ....

Nipples   : ....

Axillae   : ....

Cardiovascular Examination

Heart   : ....

Heart sound   : ....

Murmurs   : ....

Carotid pulse   : ....

Apical pulse   : ....

Peripheral pulses   : ....

Blood pressure   : ....

Abdominal Examinations

Contour   : ....

Skin   : ....

Bowel sounds   : ....

On percussion   : ....

Palpation   : ....

Musculoskeletal Examination

Back   : ....

Vertebral column alignment   : ....

Range of motion   : ....

Extremities   : ....

Lower extremities   : ....

Genitourinary and Rectum

Rectum   : ....

Female genitalia   : ....

Male genitalia   : ....

Neurological Examination

Describes tics, twitches, paresthesias   : ....

Gait   : ....

Cranial nerves   : ....

Reflexes   : ....

Co-ordination   : ....

Mental Status Examination

Level of alertness   : ....

Orientation   : ....

Memory   : ....

Language and speech   : ....

Responsiveness   : ....

Knowledge test : ....

Thinking : ....

Judgment : ....

Insight : ....

Investigation

Sl. No.	Name of investigation	Client's value	Normal value	Remarks
1.				
2.				
3.				
4.				
5.				
6.				
7.				
8.				
9.				
10.				

Treatment/Medications

Sl. No.	Name of drug	Dosage	Frequency	Class of drug
1.				
2.				
3.				
4.				
5.				
6.				
7.				
8.				
9.				
10.				

Nursing diagnosis: List down the nursing diagnosis based on needs and problems of the client with priority [Maslow's hierarchy].

Care plan: Prepare the plan of care with priority [at least 5 need-based care to be given].

Assessment	Diagnosis	Objectives	Intervention	Rationale	Evaluation

Assessment	Diagnosis	Objectives	Intervention	Rationale	Evaluation

Health education: List down the health education topics, prepare AV aids and impart the education.

Nursing Care Plan 4

HISTORY TAKING

I. Identification data:

a. Name : ....

b. Address : ....

c. Age : ....

d. Sex : ....

e. Marital status : ....

f. Education : ....

g. Occupation : ....

h. Income : ....

i. Religion : ....

j. IP No. : ....

k. Diagnosis : ....

l. Date of admission : ....

II. Presenting chief complaints: [Write down the client's problem as per their verbatim in chronological order.]

_____

_____

_____

III. History of present illness: Explain the client's problem with aggravating factors, relieving factor, precipitating factors, its characteristics, intensity, etc.

_____

_____

_____

_____

_____

_____

IV. **Past history of illness:** Explain the past medical, surgical history with its treatment, etc.

_____
_____
_____
_____
_____
_____
_____

V. **Family history:** [Family structure/family health history/social support system, etc.]

Index	
⊘	Client
◯	Female
☐	Male

Sl. No.	Name of the family members	Relationship with patient	Age/sex	Educational status	Occupational status	Marital status	Health status
1.							
2.							
3.							
4.							
5.							
6.							
7.							
8.							
9.							
10.							

VI. **Personal history:** [Bowel, bladder, sleep, diet, habit, etc.]

_____
_____
_____
_____
_____
_____
_____

PHYSICAL EXAMINATION

General Appearance

Level of consciousness : ....

Activity : ....

Body built : ....

Height : ....

Weight : ....

General grooming : ....

Body language : ....

Other observations : ....

Skin

Colour and vascularity : ....

Turgor and mobility : ....

Temperature and moisture : ....

Texture : ....

Nails : ....

Body hair growth : ....

Skin integrity : ....

Lesions : ....

Head

Shape : ....

Face : ....

Sensation : ....

Hair : ....

Condition of the scalp : ....

Facial puffiness : ....

Eyes

Eyebrows : ....

Eyelashes : ....

Eyelids : ....

Shape and appearance : ....

Sclera : ....

conjunctiva : ....

Iris : ....

Cornea : ....

Pupils : ....

Visual field : ....

Vision : ....

Use of glasses : ....

Ears

Pinnae : ....

Level in relation to eyes : ....

Canal : ....

Cilia : ....

Cerumen : ....

Tympanic membrane : ....

Hearing (audition) : ....

Tuning fork test : ....

Weber test : ....

Rinne test : ....

Hearing aid : ....

Nose and Sinuses

Size and shape : ....

Nasal septum : ....

Nasal mucosa and turbinate : ....

Patency of nares : ....

Olfactory : ....

Sinuses : ....

Mouth and Pharynx

Lips : ....

Teeth : ....

Dental caries and fillings : ....

Dental hygiene : ....

Breath odor : ....

Gums : ....

Facial and glossopharyngeal
nerve : ....

Tongue : ....

Hypoglossal : ....

Mucosa : ....

Palate : ....

Uvula : ....

Pharynx : ....

Tonsils : ....

Temporomandibular joint : ....

Neck

Appearance : ....

Thyroid : ....

Trachea : ....

Lymph nodes : ....

Thorax and Lungs

Respiratory rate : ....

Thoracic cage shape : ....

Configuration : ....

Skin color and condition : ....

Chest examination : ....

Posterior thorax : ....

Percussion of lung field : ....

Diaphragmatic exertion : ....

Lung auscultation : ....

Breath sound : ....

Respiratory pattern

Breast and Axillae

Male breasts : ....

Female breasts : ....

Nipples : ....

Axillae : ....

Cardiovascular Examination

Heart : ....

Heart sound : ....

Murmurs : ....

Carotid pulse : ....

Apical pulse : ....

Peripheral pulses : ....

Blood pressure : ....

Abdominal Examinations

Contour : ....

Skin : ....

Bowel sounds : ....

On percussion : ....

Palpation : ....

Musculoskeletal Examination

Back : ....

Vertebral column alignment : ....

Range of motion : ....

Extremities : ....

Lower extremities : ....

Genitourinary and Rectum

Rectum : ....

Female genitalia : ....

Male genitalia : ....

Neurological Examination

Describes tics,
twitches, paresthesias : ....

Gait : ....

Cranial nerves : ....

Reflexes : ....

Co-ordination : ....

Mental Status Examination

Level of alertness : ....

Orientation : ....

Memory : ....

Language and speech : ....

Responsiveness : ....

Knowledge test   : ....

Thinking   : ....

Judgment   : ....

Insight   : ....

Investigation

Sl. No.	Name of investigation	Client's value	Normal value	Remarks
1.				
2.				
3.				
4.				
5.				
6.				
7.				
8.				
9.				
10.				

Treatment/Medications

Sl. No.	Name of drug	Dosage	Frequency	Class of drug
1.				
2.				
3.				
4.				
5.				
6.				
7.				
8.				
9.				
10.				

Nursing diagnosis: List down the nursing diagnosis based on needs and problems of the client with priority [Maslow's hierarchy].

Care plan: Prepare the plan of care with priority [at least 5 need-based care to be given].

Assessment	Diagnosis	Objectives	Intervention	Rationale	Evaluation

Assessment	Diagnosis	Objectives	Intervention	Rationale	Evaluation

Health education: List down the health education topics, prepare AV aids and impart the education.

Nursing Care Plan 5

HISTORY TAKING

I. Identification data:

a. Name : ....

b. Address : ....

c. Age : ....

d. Sex : ....

e. Marital status : ....

f. Education : ....

g. Occupation : ....

h. Income : ....

i. Religion : ....

j. IP No. : ....

k. Diagnosis : ....

l. Date of admission : ....

II. Presenting chief complaints: [Write down the client's problem as per their verbatim in chronological order.]

_____

_____

_____

III. History of present illness: Explain the client's problem with aggravating factors, relieving factor, precipitating factors, its characteristics, intensity, etc.

_____

_____

_____

_____

_____

_____

37

IV. **Past history of illness:** Explain the past medical, surgical history with its treatment, etc.

_____

_____

_____

_____

_____

_____

V. **Family history:** [Family structure/family health history/social support system, etc.]

Index	
⊘	Client
○	Female
□	Male

Sl. No.	Name of the family members	Relationship with patient	Age/sex	Educational status	Occupational status	Marital status	Health status
1.							
2.							
3.							
4.							
5.							
6.							
7.							
8.							
9.							
10.							

VI. **Personal history:** [Bowel, bladder, sleep, diet, habit, etc.]

_____

_____

_____

_____

_____

_____

_____

PHYSICAL EXAMINATION

General Appearance

Level of consciousness   : ....

Activity   : ....

Body built   : ....

Height   : ....

Weight   : ....

General grooming   : ....

Body language   : ....

Other observations   : ....

Skin

Colour and vascularity   : ....

Turgor and mobility   : ....

Temperature and moisture   : ....

Texture   : ....

Nails   : ....

Body hair growth   : ....

Skin integrity   : ....

Lesions   : ....

Head

Shape   : ....

Face   : ....

Sensation   : ....

Hair   : ....

Condition of the scalp   : ....

Facial puffiness   : ....

Eyes

Eyebrows   : ....

Eyelashes   : ....

Eyelids   : ....

Shape and appearance   : ....

Sclera   : ....

conjunctiva   : ....

Iris   : ....

Cornea   : ....

Pupils   : ....

Visual field   : ....

Vision   : ....

Use of glasses   : ....

Ears

Pinnae   : ....

Level in relation to eyes   : ....

Canal   : ....

Cilia   : ....

Cerumen   : ....

Tympanic membrane   : ....

Hearing (audition)   : ....

Tuning fork test   : ....

Weber test   : ....

Rinne test   : ....

Hearing aid   : ....

Nose and Sinuses

Size and shape   : ....

Nasal septum   : ....

Nasal mucosa and turbinate   : ....

Patency of nares   : ....

Olfactory   : ....

Sinuses   : ....

Mouth and Pharynx

Lips   : ....

Teeth   : ....

Dental caries and fillings   : ....

Dental hygiene   : ....

Breath odor   : ....

Gums   : ....

Facial and glossopharyngeal
nerve   : ....

Tongue   : ....

Hypoglossal   : ....

Mucosa   : ....

Palate   : ....

Uvula   : ....

Pharynx   : ....

Tonsils   : ....

Temporomandibular joint   : ....

Neck

Appearance   : ....

Thyroid   : ....

Trachea   : ....

Lymph nodes   : ....

Thorax and Lungs

Respiratory rate   : ....

Thoracic cage shape   : ....

Configuration   : ....

Skin color and condition   : ....

Chest examination   : ....

Posterior thorax   : ....

Percussion of lung field   : ....

Diaphragmatic exertion   : ....

Lung auscultation   : ....

Breath sound   : ....

Respiratory pattern

Breast and Axillae

Male breasts   : ....

Female breasts   : ....

Nipples   : ....

Axillae   : ....

Cardiovascular Examination

Heart   : ....

Heart sound   : ....

Murmurs   : ....

Carotid pulse   : ....

Apical pulse   : ....

Peripheral pulses   : ....

Blood pressure   : ....

Abdominal Examinations

Contour : ....

Skin : ....

Bowel sounds : ....

On percussion : ....

Palpation : ....

Musculoskeletal Examination

Back : ....

Vertebral column alignment : ....

Range of motion : ....

Extremities : ....

Lower extremities : ....

Genitourinary and Rectum

Rectum : ....

Female genitalia : ....

Male genitalia : ....

Neurological Examination

Describes tics,
twitches, parasthesias : ....

Gait : ....

Cranial nerves : ....

Reflexes : ....

Co-ordinarion : ....

Mental Status Examination

Level of alertness : ....

Orientation : ....

Memory : ....

Language and speech : ....

Responsiveness : ....

Knowledge test   : ....

Thinking   : ....

Judgment   : ....

Insight   : ....

Investigation

Sl. No.	Name of investigation	Client's value	Normal value	Remarks
1.				
2.				
3.				
4.				
5.				
6.				
7.				
8.				
9.				
10.				

Treatment/Medications

Sl. No.	Name of drug	Dosage	Frequency	Class of drug
1.				
2.				
3.				
4.				
5.				
6.				
7.				
8.				
9.				
10.				

Nursing diagnosis: List down the nursing diagnosis based on needs and problems of the client with priority [Maslow's hierarchy].

Care plan: Prepare the plan of care with priority [at least 5 need-based care to be given].

Assessment	Diagnosis	Objectives	Intervention	Rationale	Evaluation

Assessment	Diagnosis	Objectives	Intervention	Rationale	Evaluation

Health education: List down the health education topics, prepare AV aids and impart the education.

Nursing Care Study/Presentation 1

I. Identification data:

a. Name : ....

b. Address : ....

c. Age : ....

d. Sex : ....

e. Marital status : ....

f. Education : ....

g. Occupation : ....

h. Income : ....

i. Religion : ....

j. IP No. : ....

k. Diagnosis : ....

l. Date of admission : ....

II. Reason for selection of the study: [Give brief description.]

_____

_____

_____

_____

_____

III. Presenting chief complaints: [Write down the client's problem as per their verbatim in chronological order.]

_____

_____

_____

_____

_____

IV. **History of present illness:** Explain the client's problem with aggravating factors, relieving factor, precipitating factors, its characteristics, intensity, etc.

_____

_____

_____

_____

_____

_____

V. **Past history of illness:** Explain the past medical, surgical history with its treatment, etc.

_____

_____

_____

_____

_____

_____

_____

VI. **Family history:** [Family structure/family health history/social support system, etc.]

_____

_____

_____

_____

_____

_____

_____

Index	
⊘	Client
◯	Female
▢	Male

Sl. No.	Name of the family members	Relationship with patient	Age/sex	Educational status	Occupational status	Marital status	Health status
1.							
2.							
3.							
4.							
5.							
6.							
7.							
8.							
9.							
10.							

VII. **Personal history:** [Bowel, bladder, sleep, diet, habit, etc.]

_____

_____

_____

_____

_____

_____

PHYSICAL EXAMINATION

General Appearance

Level of consciousness   : ....

Vital signs   : ....

    • Temp   : ....

    • Pulse   : ....

    • Respiration   : ....

    • Blood pressure   : ....

Body built   : ....

Height   : ....

Weight   : ....

General grooming   : ....

Body language   : ....

Other observations   : ....

Skin

Color and vascularity   : ....

Skin turgor   : ....

Texture and integrity   : ....

Nails   : ....

Head

Shape   : ....

Hair   : ....

Condition of the scalp   : ....

Facial puffiness   : ....

Eyes

Eyebrows, lashes, lids   : ....

Shape and appearance   : ....

Sclera   : ....

conjunctiva   : ....

Iris   : ....

Cornea   : ....

Pupils   : ....

Use of glasses   : ....

Ears

Pinnae   : ....

Level in relation to eyes   : ....

Canal   : ....

Cilia   : ....

Cerumen   : ....

Hearing aid   : ....

Nose and Sinuses

Size and shape   : ....

Nasal septum   : ....

Nasal mucosa and turbinate   : ....

Sinuses   : ....

Mouth and Pharynx

Lips   : ....

Teeth   : ....

Dental caries and fillings : ....

Dental hygiene : ....

Breath odor : ....

Gums : ....

Tongue : ....

Mucosa : ....

Palate : ....

Uvula : ....

Pharynx : ....

Tonsils : ....

Temporomandibular joint : ....

Neck

Appearance : ....

Thyroid : ....

Trachea : ....

Lymph nodes : ....

Thorax and Lungs

Respiratory rate : ....

Thoracic cage shape : ....

Posterior thorax : ....

Percussion of lung field : ....

Lung auscultation : ....

Breath sound

Respiratory pattern : ....

Breast and Axillae

Male breasts : ....

Female breasts : ....

Nipples : ....

Axillae : ....

Cardiovascular Examination

Heart : ....

Heart sound : ....

Carotid pulse : ....

Apical pulse : ....

Peripheral pulses : ....

Abdominal Examinations

Contour : ....

Skin : ....

Bowel sounds : ....

Percussion : ....

Palpation : ....

Musculoskeletal Examination

Back : ....

Vertebral column alignment : ....

Range of motion : ....

Upper extremities : ....

Lower extremities : ....

Genitourinary and Rectum

Rectum : ....

Female genitalia : ....

Male genitalia : ....

Neurological Examination

Describes tics, twitches, paresthesias : ....

Gait : ....

Cranial nerves : ....

Reflexes : ....

Co-ordination : ....

Mental Status Examination

Level of alertness : ....

Orientation : ....

Memory : ....

Language and speech : ....

Responsiveness : ....

Knowledge test : ....

Thinking : ....

Judgment : ....

Insight : ....

DESCRIPTION OF PRESENT DISEASE

Introduction

_____

_____

_____

_____

_____

Definition

_____

_____

_____

_____

_____

Related anatomy and physiology: [Give brief note.]

_____

_____

_____

_____

_____

Etiology/risk factors: [Mention present causes, possible causes and risk factors and compare with book picture.]

_____

_____

_____

_____

Pathophysiology: [Mention present pathophysiology of the patient and compared with book picture.]

_____

_____

_____

_____

_____

Clinical Manifestations

Signs and symptoms of the patient	Book picture

Investigation

Sl. No.	Name of investigation	Client's value	Normal value	Remarks
1.				
2.				
3.				
4.				
5.				
6.				
7.				
8.				
9.				
10.				

Treatment/Medications

Sl. No.	Name of drug	Dosage	Route	Frequency	Side effects	Nurses responsibilities
1.						
2.						
3.						
4.						
5.						
6.						
7.						
8.						
9.						
10.						

Nursing diagnosis: List down the nursing diagnosis based on needs and problems of the client with priority [Maslow's hierarchy].

Care plan: Prepare the plan of care with priority [at least 5 need-based care to be given].

Assessment	Diagnosis	Objectives	Intervention	Rationale	Evaluation

Assessment	Diagnosis	Objectives	Intervention	Rationale	Evaluation

Health education: List down the health education topics, prepare AV aids and impart the education.

Final impression and suspected illness/disease [states the problems or nursing diagnosis]

_____

_____

_____

_____

_____

_____

_____

Summary and Conclusion

_____

_____

_____

_____

_____

_____

_____

Bibliography

_____

_____

_____

_____

_____

_____

_____

Nursing Care Study/Presentation 2

I. Identification data:

a. Name : ....

b. Address : ....

c. Age : ....

d. Sex : ....

e. Marital status : ....

f. Education : ....

g. Occupation : ....

h. Income : ....

i. Religion : ....

j. IP No. : ....

k. Diagnosis : ....

l. Date of admission : ....

II. Reason for selection of the study: [Give brief description.]

_____

_____

_____

_____

_____

III. Presenting chief complaints: [Write down the client's problem as per their verbatim in chronological order.]

_____

_____

_____

_____

_____

IV. **History of present illness:** Explain the client's problem with aggravating factors, relieving factor, precipitating factors, its characteristics, intensity, etc.

_____

_____

_____

_____

_____

_____

V. **Past history of illness:** Explain the past medical, surgical history with its treatment, etc.

_____

_____

_____

_____

_____

_____

_____

VI. **Family history:** [Family structure/family health history/social support system, etc.]

_____

_____

_____

_____

_____

_____

_____

_____

Index	
⊘	Client
◯	Female
☐	Male

Sl. No.	Name of the family members	Relationship with patient	Age/sex	Educational status	Occupational status	Marital status	Health status
1.							
2.							
3.							
4.							
5.							
6.							
7.							
8.							
9.							
10.							

VII. **Personal history:** [Bowel, bladder, sleep, diet, habit, etc.]

_____

_____

_____

_____

_____

_____

_____

PHYSICAL EXAMINATION

General Appearance

Level of consciousness : ....

Vital signs : ....

• Temp : ....

• Pulse : ....

• Respiration : ....

• Blood pressure : ....

Body built : ....

Height : ....

Weight : ....

General grooming : ....

Body language : ....

Other observations : ....

Skin

Color and vascularity : ....

Skin turgor : ....

Texture and integrity : ....

Nails : ....

Head

Shape : ....

Hair : ....

Condition of the scalp : ....

Facial puffiness : ....

Eyes

Eyebrows, lashes, lids : ....

Shape and appearance : ....

Sclera : ....

conjunctiva : ....

Iris : ....

Cornea : ....

Pupils : ....

Use of glasses : ....

Ears

Pinnae : ....

Level in relation to eyes : ....

Canal : ....

Cilia : ....

Cerumen : ....

Hearing aid : ....

Nose and Sinuses

Size and shape : ....

Nasal septum : ....

Nasal mucosa and turbinate : ....

Sinuses : ....

Mouth and Pharynx

Lips : ....

Teeth : ....

Dental caries and fillings : ....

Dental hygiene : ....

Breath odor : ....

Gums : ....

Tongue : ....

Mucosa : ....

Palate : ....

Uvula : ....

Pharynx : ....

Tonsils : ....

Temporomandibular joint : ....

Neck

Appearance : ....

Thyroid : ....

Trachea : ....

Lymph nodes : ....

Thorax and Lungs

Respiratory rate : ....

Thoracic cage shape : ....

Posterior thorax : ....

Percussion of lung field : ....

Lung auscultation : ....

Breath sound

Respiratory pattern : ....

Breast and Axillae

Male breasts : ....

Female breasts : ....

Nipples : ....

Axillae : ....

Cardiovascular Examination

Heart : ....

Heart sound : ....

Carotid pulse : ....

Apical pulse : ....

Peripheral pulses : ....

Abdominal Examinations

Contour : ....

Skin : ....

Bowel sounds : ....

Percussion : ....

Palpation : ....

Musculoskeletal Examination

Back : ....

Vertebral column alignment : ....

Range of motion : ....

Upper extremities : ....

Lower extremities : ....

Genitourinary and Rectum

Rectum : ....

Female genitalia : ....

Male genitalia : ....

Neurological Examination

Describes tics, twitches, paresthesias : ....

Gait : ....

Cranial nerves : ....

Reflexes : ....

Co-ordination : ....

Mental Status Examination

Level of alertness : ....

Orientation : ....

Memory : ....

Language and speech : ....

Responsiveness : ....

Knowledge test : ....

Thinking : ....

Judgment : ....

Insight : ....

DESCRIPTION OF PRESENT DISEASE

Introduction

_____
_____
_____
_____
_____

Definition

_____
_____
_____
_____
_____

Related anatomy and physiology: [Give brief note.]

_____
_____
_____
_____
_____

Etiology/risk factors [Mention present causes, possible causes and risk factors and compare with book picture.]

_____
_____
_____
_____

Pathophysiology: [Mention present pathophysiology of the patient and compared with book picture.]

_____
_____
_____
_____

Clinical Manifestations

Signs and symptoms of the patient	Book picture

Investigation

Sl. No.	Name of investigation	Client's value	Normal value	Remarks
1.				
2.				
3.				
4.				
5.				
6.				
7.				
8.				
9.				
10.				

Treatment/Medications

Sl. No.	Name of drug	Dosage	Route	Frequency	Side effects	Nurses responsibilities
1.						
2.						
3.						
4.						
5.						
6.						
7.						
8.						
9.						
10.						

Nursing diagnosis: List down the nursing diagnosis based on needs and problems of the client with priority [Maslow's hierarchy].

Care plan: Prepare the plan of care with priority [at least 5 need-based care to be given].

Assessment	Diagnosis	Objectives	Intervention	Rationale	Evaluation

Assessment	Diagnosis	Objectives	Intervention	Rationale	Evaluation

Health education: List down the health education topics, prepare AV aids and impart the education.

Final impression and suspected illness/disease [states the problems or nursing diagnosis]

_____
_____
_____
_____
_____
_____
_____
_____
_____

Summary and Conclusion

_____
_____
_____
_____
_____
_____
_____
_____
_____

Bibliography

_____
_____
_____
_____
_____
_____
_____
_____

Nursing Care Study/Presentation 3

I. Identification data:

a. Name   : ....

b. Address   : ....

c. Age   : ....

d. Sex   : ....

e. Marital status   : ....

f. Education   : ....

g. Occupation   : ....

h. Income   : ....

i. Religion   : ....

j. IP No.   : ....

k. Diagnosis   : ....

l. Date of admission : ....

II. Reason for selection of the study: [Give brief description.]

_____

_____

_____

_____

_____

III. Presenting chief complaints: [Write down the client's problem as per their verbatim in chronological order.]

_____

_____

_____

_____

_____

IV. **History of present illness:** Explain the client's problem with aggravating factors, relieving factor, precipitating factors, its characteristics, intensity, etc.

_____

_____

_____

_____

_____

_____

V. **Past history of illness:** Explain the past medical, surgical history with its treatment, etc.

_____

_____

_____

_____

_____

_____

_____

VI. **Family history:** [Family structure/family health history/social support system, etc.]

_____

_____

_____

_____

_____

_____

_____

Index	
⊘	Client
◯	Female
▢	Male

Sl. No.	Name of the family members	Relationship with patient	Age/sex	Educational status	Occupational status	Marital status	Health status
1.							
2.							
3.							
4.							
5.							
6.							
7.							
8.							
9.							
10.							

VII. **Personal history:** [Bowel, bladder, sleep, diet, habit, etc.]

_____

_____

_____

_____

_____

_____

_____

PHYSICAL EXAMINATION

General Appearance

Level of consciousness   : ....

Vital signs   : ....

  • Temp   : ....

  • Pulse   : ....

  • Respiration   : ....

  • Blood pressure   : ....

Body built   : ....

Height   : ....

Weight   : ....

General grooming   : ....

Body language   : ....

Other observations   : ....

Skin

Color and vascularity : ....

Skin turgor : ....

Texture and integrity : ....

Nails : ....

Head

Shape : ....

Hair : ....

Condition of the scalp : ....

Facial puffiness : ....

Eyes

Eyebrows, lashes, lids : ....

Shape and appearance : ....

Sclera : ....

conjunctiva : ....

Iris : ....

Cornea : ....

Pupils : ....

Use of glasses : ....

Ears

Pinnae : ....

Level in relation to eyes : ....

Canal : ....

Cilia : ....

Cerumen : ....

Hearing aid : ....

Nose and Sinuses

Size and shape : ....

Nasal septum : ....

Nasal mucosa and turbinate : ....

Sinuses : ....

Mouth and Pharynx

Lips : ....

Teeth : ....

Dental caries and fillings : ....

Dental hygiene : ....

Breath odor : ....

Gums : ....

Tongue : ....

Mucosa : ....

Palate : ....

Uvula : ....

Pharynx : ....

Tonsils : ....

Temporomandibular joint : ....

Neck

Appearance : ....

Thyroid : ....

Trachea : ....

Lymph nodes : ....

Thorax and Lungs

Respiratory rate : ....

Thoracic cage shape : ....

Posterior thorax : ....

Percussion of lung field : ....

Lung auscultation : ....

Breath sound

Respiratory pattern : ....

Breast and Axillae

Male breasts : ....

Female breasts : ....

Nipples : ....

Axillae : ....

Cardiovascular Examination

Heart : ....

Heart sound : ....

Carotid pulse : ....

Apical pulse : ....

Peripheral pulses : ....

Abdominal Examinations

Contour   : ....

Skin   : ....

Bowel sounds   : ....

Percussion   : ....

Palpation   : ....

Musculoskeletal Examination

Back   : ....

Vertebral column alignment : ....

Range of motion   : ....

Upper extremities   : ....

Lower extremities   : ....

Genitourinary and Rectum

Rectum   : ....

Female genitalia   : ....

Male genitalia   : ....

Neurological Examination

Describes tics, twitches, paresthesias   : ....

Gait   : ....

Cranial nerves   : ....

Reflexes   : ....

Co-ordination   : ....

Mental Status Examination

Level of alertness   : ....

Orientation   : ....

Memory   : ....

Language and speech : ....

Responsiveness   : ....

Knowledge test   : ....

Thinking   : ....

Judgment   : ....

Insight   : ....

DESCRIPTION OF PRESENT DISEASE

Introduction

_____

_____

_____

_____

_____

Definition

_____

_____

_____

_____

_____

Related anatomy and physiology: [Give brief note.]

_____

_____

_____

_____

_____

Etiology/risk factors: [Mention present causes, possible causes and risk factors and compare with book picture.]

_____

_____

_____

_____

Pathophysiology: [Mention present pathophysiology of the patient and compared with book picture.]

_____

_____

_____

_____

_____

Clinical Manifestations

Signs and symptoms of the patient	Book picture

Investigation

Sl. No.	Name of investigation	Client's value	Normal value	Remarks
1.				
2.				
3.				
4.				
5.				
6.				
7.				
8.				
9.				
10.				

Treatment/Medications

Sl. No.	Name of drug	Dosage	Route	Frequency	Side effects	Nurses responsibilities
1.						
2.						
3.						
4.						
5.						
6.						
7.						
8.						
9.						
10.						

Nursing diagnosis: List down the nursing diagnosis based on needs and problems of the client with priority [Maslow's hierarchy].

Care plan: Prepare the plan of care with priority [at least 5 need-based care to be given].

Assessment	Diagnosis	Objectives	Intervention	Rationale	Evaluation

Assessment	Diagnosis	Objectives	Intervention	Rationale	Evaluation

Health education: List down the health education topics, prepare AV aids and impart the education.

Final impression and suspected illness/disease [states the problems or nursing diagnosis]

_____
_____
_____
_____
_____
_____
_____
_____

Summary and Conclusion

_____
_____
_____
_____
_____
_____
_____
_____
_____

Bibliography

_____
_____
_____
_____
_____
_____

Nursing Care Study/Presentation 4

I. Identification data:

a. Name : ....

b. Address : ....

c. Age : ....

d. Sex : ....

e. Marital status : ....

f. Education : ....

g. Occupation : ....

h. Income : ....

i. Religion : ....

j. IP No. : ....

k. Diagnosis : ....

l. Date of admission : ....

II. Reason for selection of the study: [Give brief description.]

_____

_____

_____

_____

_____

III. Presenting chief complaints: [Write down the client's problem as per their verbatim in chronological order.]

_____

_____

_____

_____

_____

IV. **History of present illness:** Explain the client's problem with aggravating factors, relieving factor, precipitating factors, its characteristics, intensity, etc.

_____
_____
_____
_____
_____
_____

V. **Past history of illness:** Explain the past medical, surgical history with its treatment, etc.

_____
_____
_____
_____
_____
_____
_____

VI. **Family history:** [Family structure/family health history/social support system, etc.]

_____
_____
_____
_____
_____
_____
_____

Index	
⊘	Client
◯	Female
□	Male

Sl. No.	Name of the family members	Relationship with patient	Age/sex	Educational status	Occupational status	Marital status	Health status
1.							
2.							
3.							
4.							
5.							
6.							
7.							
8.							
9.							
10.							

VII. **Personal history:** [Bowel, bladder, sleep, diet, habit, etc.]

_____

_____

_____

_____

_____

_____

_____

PHYSICAL EXAMINATION

General Appearance

Level of consciousness   : ....

Vital signs   : ....

  • Temp   : ....

  • Pulse   : ....

  • Respiration   : ....

  • Blood pressure   : ....

Body built   : ....

Height   : ....

Weight   : ....

General grooming   : ....

Body language   : ....

Other observations   : ....

Skin

Color and vascularity : ....

Skin turgor : ....

Texture and integrity : ....

Nails : ....

Head

Shape : ....

Hair : ....

Condition of the scalp : ....

Facial puffiness : ....

Eyes

Eyebrows, lashes, lids : ....

Shape and appearance : ....

Sclera : ....

conjunctiva : ....

Iris : ....

Cornea : ....

Pupils : ....

Use of glasses : ....

Ears

Pinnae : ....

Level in relation to eyes : ....

Canal : ....

Cilia : ....

Cerumen : ....

Hearing aid : ....

Nose and Sinuses

Size and shape : ....

Nasal septum : ....

Nasal mucosa and turbinate : ....

Sinuses : ....

Mouth and Pharynx

Lips : ....

Teeth : ....

Dental caries and fillings : ....
Dental hygiene : ....
Breath odor : ....
Gums : ....
Tongue : ....
Mucosa : ....
Palate : ....
Uvula : ....
Pharynx : ....
Tonsils : ....
Temporomandibular joint : ....

Neck
Appearance : ....
Thyroid : ....
Trachea : ....
Lymph nodes : ....

Thorax and Lungs
Respiratory rate : ....
Thoracic cage shape : ....
Posterior thorax : ....
Percussion of lung field : ....
Lung auscultation : ....
Breath sound
Respiratory pattern : ....

Breast and Axillae
Male breasts : ....
Female breasts : ....
Nipples : ....
Axillae : ....

Cardiovascular Examination
Heart : ....
Heart sound : ....
Carotid pulse : ....
Apical pulse : ....
Peripheral pulses : ....

Abdominal Examinations

Contour : ....

Skin : ....

Bowel sounds : ....

Percussion : ....

Palpation : ....

Musculoskeletal Examination

Back : ....

Vertebral column alignment : ....

Range of motion : ....

Upper extremities : ....

Lower extremities : ....

Genitourinary and Rectum

Rectum : ....

Female genitalia : ....

Male genitalia : ....

Neurological Examination

Describes tics, twitches, paresthesias : ....

Gait : ....

Cranial nerves : ....

Reflexes : ....

Co-ordination : ....

Mental Status Examination

Level of alertness : ....

Orientation : ....

Memory : ....

Language and speech : ....

Responsiveness : ....

Knowledge test : ....

Thinking : ....

Judgment : ....

Insight : ....

DESCRIPTION OF PRESENT DISEASE

Introduction

_____
_____
_____
_____
_____

Definition

_____
_____
_____
_____

Related anatomy and physiology: [Give brief note.]

_____
_____
_____
_____
_____

Etiology/risk factors: [Mention present causes, possible causes and risk factors and compare with book picture.]

_____
_____
_____
_____

Pathophysiology: [Mention present pathophysiology of the patient and compared with book picture.]

_____
_____
_____
_____

Clinical Manifestations

Signs and symptoms of the patient	Book picture

Investigation

Sl. No.	Name of investigation	Client's value	Normal value	Remarks
1.				
2.				
3.				
4.				
5.				
6.				
7.				
8.				
9.				
10.				

Treatment/Medications

Sl. No.	Name of drug	Dosage	Route	Frequency	Side effects	Nurses responsibilities
1.						
2.						
3.						
4.						
5.						
6.						
7.						
8.						
9.						
10.						

Nursing diagnosis: List down the nursing diagnosis based on needs and problems of the client with priority [Maslow's hierarchy].

Care plan: Prepare the plan of care with priority [at least 5 need-based care to be given].

Assessment	Diagnosis	Objectives	Intervention	Rationale	Evaluation

Assessment	Diagnosis	Objectives	Intervention	Rationale	Evaluation

Health education: List down the health education topics, prepare AV aids and impart the education.

Final impression and suspected illness/disease [states the problems or nursing diagnosis]

_____
_____
_____
_____
_____
_____
_____

Summary and Conclusion

_____
_____
_____
_____
_____
_____
_____

Bibliography

_____
_____
_____
_____
_____
_____

Nursing Care Study/Presentation 5

I. Identification data:

   a. Name   : ....

   b. Address   : ....

   c. Age   : ....

   d. Sex   : ....

   e. Marital status : ....

   f. Education   : ....

   g. Occupation : ....

   h. Income   : ....

   i. Religion   : ....

   j. IP No.   : ....

   k. Diagnosis   : ....

   l. Date of admission : ....

II. Reason for selection of the study: [Give brief description.]

_____

_____

_____

_____

_____

III. Presenting chief complaints: [Write down the client's problem as per their verbatim in chronological order.]

_____

_____

_____

_____

_____

IV. **History of present illness:** Explain the client's problem with aggravating factors, relieving factor, precipitating factors, its characteristics, intensity, etc.

_____

_____

_____

_____

_____

_____

V. **Past history of illness:** Explain the past medical, surgical history with its treatment, etc.

_____

_____

_____

_____

_____

_____

_____

VI. **Family history:** [Family structure/family health history/social support system, etc.]

_____

_____

_____

_____

_____

_____

_____

Index	
⊘	Client
◯	Female
▢	Male

Sl. No.	Name of the family members	Relationship with patient	Age/sex	Educational status	Occupational status	Marital status	Health status
1.							
2.							
3.							
4.							
5.							
6.							
7.							
8.							
9.							
10.							

VII. **Personal history:** [Bowel, bladder, sleep, diet, habit, etc.]

_____

_____

_____

_____

_____

_____

_____

PHYSICAL EXAMINATION

General Appearance

Level of consciousness   : ....

Vital signs   : ....

   • Temp   : ....

   • Pulse   : ....

   • Respiration   : ....

   • Blood pressure   : ....

Body built   : ....

Height   : ....

Weight   : ....

General grooming   : ....

Body language   : ....

Other observations   : ....

Skin

Color and vascularity : ....

Skin turgor : ....

Texture and integrity : ....

Nails : ....

Head

Shape : ....

Hair : ....

Condition of the scalp : ....

Facial puffiness : ....

Eyes

Eyebrows, lashes, lids : ....

Shape and appearance : ....

Sclera : ....

conjunctiva : ....

Iris : ....

Cornea : ....

Pupils : ....

Use of glasses : ....

Ears

Pinnae : ....

Level in relation to eyes : ....

Canal : ....

Cilia : ....

Cerumen : ....

Hearing aid : ....

Nose and Sinuses

Size and shape : ....

Nasal septum : ....

Nasal mucosa and turbinate : ....

Sinuses : ....

Mouth and Pharynx

Lips : ....

Teeth : ....

Dental caries and fillings : ....

Dental hygiene : ....

Breath odor : ....

Gums : ....

Tongue : ....

Mucosa : ....

Palate : ....

Uvula : ....

Pharynx : ....

Tonsils : ....

Temporomandibular joint : ....

Neck

Appearance : ....

Thyroid : ....

Trachea : ....

Lymph nodes : ....

Thorax and Lungs

Respiratory rate : ....

Thoracic cage shape : ....

Posterior thorax : ....

Percussion of lung field : ....

Lung auscultation : ....

Breath sound

Respiratory pattern : ....

Breast and Axillae

Male breasts : ....

Female breasts : ....

Nipples : ....

Axillae : ....

Cardiovascular Examination

Heart : ....

Heart sound : ....

Carotid pulse : ....

Apical pulse : ....

Peripheral pulses : ....

Abdominal Examinations

Contour : ....

Skin : ....

Bowel sounds : ....

Percussion : ....

Palpation : ....

Musculoskeletal Examination

Back : ....

Vertebral column alignment : ....

Range of motion : ....

Upper extremities : ....

Lower extremities : ....

Genitourinary and Rectum

Rectum : ....

Female genitalia : ....

Male genitalia : ....

Neurological Examination

Describes tics, twitches,
paresthesias : ....

Gait : ....

Cranial nerves : ....

Reflexes : ....

Co-ordination : ....

Mental Status Examination

Level of alertness : ....

Orientation : ....

Memory : ....

Language and speech : ....

Responsiveness : ....

Knowledge test : ....

Thinking : ....

Judgment : ....

Insight : ....

DESCRIPTION OF PRESENT DISEASE

Introduction

_____

_____

_____

_____

_____

Definition

_____

_____

_____

_____

_____

Related anatomy and physiology: [Give brief note.]

_____

_____

_____

_____

_____

Etiology/risk factors: [Mention present causes, possible causes and risk factors and compare with book picture.]

_____

_____

_____

_____

Pathophysiology: [Mention present pathophysiology of the patient and compared with book picture.]

_____

_____

_____

_____

Clinical Manifestations

Signs and symptoms of the patient	Book picture

Investigation

Sl. No.	Name of investigation	Client's value	Normal value	Remarks
1.				
2.				
3.				
4.				
5.				
6.				
7.				
8.				
9.				
10.				

Treatment/Medications

Sl. No.	Name of drug	Dosage	Route	Frequency	Side effects	Nurses responsibilities
1.						
2.						
3.						
4.						
5.						
6.						
7.						
8.						
9.						
10.						

Nursing diagnosis: List down the nursing diagnosis based on needs and problems of the client with priority [Maslow's hierarchy].

Care plan: Prepare the plan of care with priority [at least 5 need-based care to be given].

Assessment	Diagnosis	Objectives	Intervention	Rationale	Evaluation

Assessment	Diagnosis	Objectives	Intervention	Rationale	Evaluation

Health education: List down the health education topics, prepare AV aids and impart the education.

Final impression and suspected illness/disease [states the problems or nursing diagnosis]

_____

_____

_____

_____

_____

_____

_____

Summary and Conclusion

_____

_____

_____

_____

_____

_____

_____

Bibliography

_____

_____

_____

_____

_____

_____

Bedside Procedure 1

I. Identification data:

 a. Name : ....

 b. Address : ....

 c. Age : ....

 d. Sex : ....

 e. Marital status : ....

 f. Education : ....

 g. Occupation : ....

 h. Income : ....

 i. Religion : ....

 j. IP No. : ....

 k. Diagnosis : ....

 l. Date of admission : ....

II. Definition of the disease:

_____

_____

_____

_____

_____

_____

III. Nursing assessment: Mention the key points of subjective and objective data

_____

_____

_____

_____

_____

_____

IV. **Nursing diagnosis:** List of problems based on priority [Maslow's hierarchy]

1. _____
2. _____
3. _____
4. _____
5. _____
6. _____
7. _____
8. _____
9. _____
10. _____

V. **Planning:** State the objectives of the care

1. _____
2. _____
3. _____
4. _____
5. _____

VI. **Intervention:** State the interventions to be performed

1. _____
2. _____
3. _____
4. _____
5. _____

Nursing procedure: Related to client condition

- Name of the procedure   : _____
- Definition of the procedure : _____
- Purpose of the procedure   : _____

Articles Required for Procedure

1. _____
2. _____
3. _____

4. _____

5. _____

6. _____

7. _____

8. _____

9. _____

10. _____

Preparation of the Client

1. _____

2. _____

3. _____

4. _____

5. _____

6. _____

7. _____

8. _____

9. _____

10. _____

Steps of the Procedures with Rationale

Sl. No.	Steps of the procedure	Rationale
1.		
2.		
3.		
4.		
5.		
6.		
7.		
8.		
9.		
10.		
11.		
12.		

Care of the Client after Procedure

_____
_____
_____
_____
_____
_____

Care of the Articles/Area

_____
_____
_____
_____
_____

Comments

_____
_____
_____
_____
_____

Health Teaching

_____
_____
_____
_____
_____

Bedside Procedure 2

I. Identification data:

a. Name : ....

b. Address : ....

c. Age : ....

d. Sex : ....

e. Marital status : ....

f. Education : ....

g. Occupation : ....

h. Income : ....

i. Religion : ....

j. IP No. : ....

k. Diagnosis : ....

l. Date of admission : ....

II. Definition of the disease:

_____

_____

_____

_____

_____

_____

III. Nursing assessment: Mention the key points of subjective and objective data

_____

_____

_____

_____

_____

_____

IV. **Nursing diagnosis:** List of problems based on priority [Maslow's hierarchy]

1. _____
2. _____
3. _____
4. _____
5. _____
6. _____
7. _____
8. _____
9. _____
10. _____

V. **Planning:** State the objectives of the care

1. _____
2. _____
3. _____
4. _____
5. _____

VI. **Intervention:** State the interventions to be performed

1. _____
2. _____
3. _____
4. _____
5. _____

Nursing procedure: Related to client condition

• Name of the procedure   : _____
• Definition of the procedure : _____
• Purpose of the procedure   : _____

Articles Required for Procedure

1. _____
2. _____
3. _____

4. _____
5. _____
6. _____
7. _____
8. _____
9. _____
10. _____

Preparation of the Client

1. _____
2. _____
3. _____
4. _____
5. _____
6. _____
7. _____
8. _____
9. _____
10. _____

Steps of the Procedures with Rationale

Sl. No.	Steps of the procedure	Rationale
1.		
2.		
3.		
4.		
5.		
6.		
7.		
8.		
9.		
10.		
11.		
12.		

Care of the Client after Procedure

_____
_____
_____
_____
_____

Care of the Articles/Area

_____
_____
_____
_____
_____

Comments

_____
_____
_____
_____
_____

Health Teaching

_____
_____
_____
_____
_____

Bedside Procedure 3

I. Identification data:

a. Name : ....

b. Address : ....

c. Age : ....

d. Sex : ....

e. Marital status : ....

f. Education : ....

g. Occupation : ....

h. Income : ....

i. Religion : ....

j. IP No. : ....

k. Diagnosis : ....

l. Date of admission : ....

II. Definition of the disease:

_____

_____

_____

_____

_____

_____

III. Nursing assessment: Mention the key points of subjective and objective data

_____

_____

_____

_____

_____

_____

IV. **Nursing diagnosis:** List of problems based on priority [Maslow's hierarchy]

1. _____
2. _____
3. _____
4. _____
5. _____
6. _____
7. _____
8. _____
9. _____
10. _____

V. **Planning:** State the objectives of the care

1. _____
2. _____
3. _____
4. _____
5. _____

VI. **Intervention:** State the interventions to be performed

1. _____
2. _____
3. _____
4. _____
5. _____

Nursing procedure: Related to client condition

- Name of the procedure   : _____
- Definition of the procedure : _____
- Purpose of the procedure   : _____

Articles Required for Procedure

1. _____
2. _____
3. _____

4. _____

5. _____

6. _____

7. _____

8. _____

9. _____

10. _____

Preparation of the Client

1. _____

2. _____

3. _____

4. _____

5. _____

6. _____

7. _____

8. _____

9. _____

10. _____

Steps of the Procedures with Rationale

Sl. No.	Steps of the procedure	Rationale
1.		
2.		
3.		
4.		
5.		
6.		
7.		
8.		
9.		
10.		
11.		
12.		

Care of the Client after Procedure

_____

_____

_____

_____

_____

Care of the Articles/Area

_____

_____

_____

_____

_____

Comments

_____

_____

_____

_____

_____

Health Teaching

_____

_____

_____

_____

_____

Bedside Procedure 4

I. Identification data:

a. Name   : ....

b. Address   : ....

c. Age   : ....

d. Sex   : ....

e. Marital status   : ....

f. Education   : ....

g. Occupation   : ....

h. Income   : ....

i. Religion   : ....

j. IP No.   : ....

k. Diagnosis   : ....

l. Date of admission : ....

II. Definition of the disease:

_____

_____

_____

_____

_____

_____

III. Nursing assessment: Mention the key points of subjective and objective data

_____

_____

_____

_____

_____

_____

IV. **Nursing diagnosis:** List of problems based on priority [Maslow's hierarchy]

1. _____
2. _____
3. _____
4. _____
5. _____
6. _____
7. _____
8. _____
9. _____
10. _____

V. **Planning:** State the objectives of the care

1. _____
2. _____
3. _____
4. _____
5. _____

VI. **Intervention:** State the interventions to be performed

1. _____
2. _____
3. _____
4. _____
5. _____

Nursing procedure: Related to client condition

- Name of the procedure   : _____
- Definition of the procedure : _____
- Purpose of the procedure   : _____

Articles Required for Procedure

1. _____
2. _____
3. _____

4. _____

5. _____

6. _____

7. _____

8. _____

9. _____

10. _____

Preparation of the Client

1. _____

2. _____

3. _____

4. _____

5. _____

6. _____

7. _____

8. _____

9. _____

10. _____

Steps of the Procedures with Rationale

Sl. No.	Steps of the procedure	Rationale
1.		
2.		
3.		
4.		
5.		
6.		
7.		
8.		
9.		
10.		
11.		
12.		

Care of the Client after Procedure

_____

_____

_____

_____

_____

Care of the Articles/Area

_____

_____

_____

_____

_____

Comments

_____

_____

_____

_____

_____

Health Teaching

_____

_____

_____

_____

Bedside Procedure 5

I. Identification data:

a. Name : ....

b. Address : ....

c. Age : ....

d. Sex : ....

e. Marital status : ....

f. Education : ....

g. Occupation : ....

h. Income : ....

i. Religion : ....

j. IP No. : ....

k. Diagnosis : ....

l. Date of admission : ....

II. Definition of the disease:

_____

_____

_____

_____

_____

_____

III. Nursing assessment: Mention the key points of subjective and objective data

_____

_____

_____

_____

_____

_____

_____

IV. **Nursing diagnosis:** List of problems based on priority [Maslow's hierarchy]

1. _____
2. _____
3. _____
4. _____
5. _____
6. _____
7. _____
8. _____
9. _____
10. _____

V. **Planning:** State the objectives of the care

1. _____
2. _____
3. _____
4. _____
5. _____

VI. **Intervention:** State the interventions to be performed

1. _____
2. _____
3. _____
4. _____
5. _____

Nursing procedure: Related to client condition

- Name of the procedure   : _____
- Definition of the procedure   : _____
- Purpose of the procedure   : _____

Articles Required for Procedure

1. _____
2. _____
3. _____

4. _____

5. _____

6. _____

7. _____

8. _____

9. _____

10. _____

Preparation of the Client

1. _____

2. _____

3. _____

4. _____

5. _____

6. _____

7. _____

8. _____

9. _____

10. _____

Steps of the Procedures with Rationale

Sl. No.	Steps of the procedure	Rationale
1.		
2.		
3.		
4.		
5.		
6.		
7.		
8.		
9.		
10.		
11.		
12.		

Care of the Client after Procedure

_____
_____
_____
_____
_____

Care of the Articles/Area

_____
_____
_____
_____
_____

Comments

_____
_____
_____
_____
_____

Health Teaching

_____
_____
_____
_____
_____

Drug Study 1

Trade name   : ....

Generic name   : ....

Drug group   : ....

Mode of action   : ....

                       : ....

                       : ....

                       : ....

Indication of drug : ....

Dosage   : ....

Route of
administration   : ....

Side effects   : ....

                       : ....

                       : ....

                       : ....

Contraindication   : ....

                       : ....

                       : ....

Nurses
responsibilities   : ....

                       : ....

                       : ....

                       : ....

                       : ....

References

_____
_____
_____
_____
_____
_____
_____
_____
_____
_____
_____

Drug Study 2

Trade name : ....

Generic name : ....

Drug group : ....

Mode of action : ....

: ....

: ....

: ....

Indication of drug : ....

Dosage : ....

Route of
administration : ....

Side effects : ....

: ....

: ....

: ....

Contraindication : ....

: ....

: ....

Nurses
responsibilities : ....

: ....

: ....

: ....

: ....

References

_____

_____

_____

_____

_____

_____

_____

_____

_____

_____

_____

Drug Study 3

Trade name   : ....

Generic name   : ....

Drug group   : ....

Mode of action   : ....

                    : ....

                    : ....

                    : ....

Indication of drug : ....

Dosage   : ....

Route of
administration   : ....

Side effects   : ....

                    : ....

                    : ....

                    : ....

Contraindication   : ....

                    : ....

                    : ....

Nurses
responsibilities   : ....

                    : ....

                    : ....

                    : ....

                    : ....

References

_____
_____
_____
_____
_____
_____
_____
_____
_____
_____
_____

Drug Study 4

Trade name   : ....

Generic name   : ....

Drug group   : ....

Mode of action : ....

                     : ....

                     : ....

                     : ....

Indication of drug : ....

Dosage   : ....

Route of
administration : ....

Side effects   : ....

                     : ....

                     : ....

                     : ....

Contraindication : ....

                     : ....

                     : ....

Nurses
responsibilities : ....

                     : ....

                     : ....

                     : ....

                     : ....

References

_____

_____

_____

_____

_____

_____

_____

_____

_____

_____

Drug Study 5

Trade name : ....

Generic name : ....

Drug group : ....

Mode of action : ....

: ....

: ....

: ....

Indication of drug : ....

Dosage : ....

Route of
administration : ....

Side effects : ....

: ....

: ....

: ....

Contraindication : ....

: ....

: ....

Nurses
responsibilities : ....

: ....

: ....

: ....

: ....

References

_____

_____

_____

_____

_____

_____

_____

_____

_____

_____

Health Talk 1

Trade name : ....

Name of student–teacher : ....

Year : ....

Subject : ....

Topic : ....

Group and size : ....

Method of teaching : ....

AV aids : ....

Date and time : ....

Duration of teaching : ....

Venue : ....

Name of the supervisor : ....

Previous knowledge of the group : ....

General Objectives

_____

_____

_____

_____

Specific Objectives

_____

_____

_____

_____

Sl. No.	Time	Objectives	Content	Teacher/learner activities	AV aids	Evaluations

Summary and Conclusion

_____

_____

_____

_____

References

_____

_____

_____

_____

_____

Health Talk 2

Trade name : ....

Name of student–teacher : ....

Year : ....

Subject : ....

Topic : ....

Group and size : ....

Method of teaching : ....

AV aids : ....

Date and time : ....

Duration of teaching : ....

Venue : ....

Name of the supervisor : ....

Previous knowledge of the group : ....

General Objectives

_____

_____

_____

_____

_____

Specific Objectives

_____

_____

_____

_____

_____

Sl. No.	Time	Objectives	Content	Teacher/learner activities	AV aids	Evaluations

Summary and Conclusion

_____

_____

_____

_____

_____

References

_____

_____

_____

_____

_____

Health Talk 3

Trade name : ....

Name of student–teacher : ....

Year : ....

Subject : ....

Topic : ....

Group and size : ....

Method of teaching : ....

AV aids : ....

Date and time : ....

Duration of teaching : ....

Venue : ....

Name of the supervisor : ....

Previous knowledge of the group : ....

General Objectives

_____

_____

_____

_____

Specific Objectives

_____

_____

_____

_____

_____

Sl. No.	Time	Objectives	Content	Teacher/learner activities	AV aids	Evaluations

Summary and Conclusion

_____

_____

_____

_____

_____

References

_____

_____

_____

_____

_____

Health Talk 4

Trade name : ....

Name of student–teacher : ....

Year : ....

Subject : ....

Topic : ....

Group and size : ....

Method of teaching : ....

AV aids : ....

Date and time : ....

Duration of teaching : ....

Venue : ....

Name of the supervisor : ....

Previous knowledge of the group : ....

General Objectives

_____

_____

_____

_____

_____

Specific Objectives

_____

_____

_____

_____

_____

Sl. No.	Time	Objectives	Content	Teacher/learner activities	AV aids	Evaluations

Summary and Conclusion

_____

_____

_____

_____

_____

References

_____

_____

_____

_____

_____

Health Talk 5

Trade name   : ....

Name of student–teacher   : ....

Year   : ....

Subject   : ....

Topic   : ....

Group and size   : ....

Method of teaching   : ....

AV aids   : ....

Date and time   : ....

Duration of teaching   : ....

Venue   : ....

Name of the supervisor   : ....

Previous knowledge of the group : ....

General Objectives

_____

_____

_____

_____

_____

Specific Objectives

_____

_____

_____

_____

_____

Sl. No.	Time	Objectives	Content	Teacher/learner activities	AV aids	Evaluations

Summary and Conclusion

_____

_____

_____

_____

_____

References

_____

_____

_____

_____

_____

Intensive Care Unit (ICU)

Report of Clinical Experience in the Intensive Care Unit

General objectives

_____
_____
_____
_____
_____
_____
_____

Principles of intensive care unit

_____
_____
_____
_____
_____
_____
_____

Physical layout of ICU [draw a diagram of ICU setup]

_____
_____
_____
_____
_____
_____

List of equipment used in ICU

Sl. No.	Name of the equipment	Purpose

List of procedures performed in ICU

Sl. No.	Name of the procedure	Purposes	Indication	Nurses responsibilities assisted/performed

Nurses responsibilities in ICU

1. _____
2. _____
3. _____

4. _____

5. _____

6. _____

7. _____

8. _____

9. _____

10. _____

Summary of student clinical experience

_____

_____

_____

_____

_____

_____

_____

_____

_____

_____

_____

Operation Theatre

Report of Clinical Experience in the Operation Theatre

General objectives

_____
_____
_____
_____
_____
_____
_____

Physical layout of operation theatre [draw diagram of OT]

_____
_____
_____
_____
_____
_____
_____

Method of Sterilization of Equipment/Linen in Operation Theatre [OT]

Sterilization

- Blunt instruments : _____
- Sharp instruments : _____
- Linen : _____
- Chemical used : _____
- Fumigation of OT : _____

Universal precautions

- Medical asepsis : _____
- Surgical asepsis : _____

Setting up of trolley for operation [general or specific]

List of articles, instruments and their purposes

Sl. No.	Name of the article	Purpose

List of surgeries witnessed or assisted

Sl. No.	Name of the client	Age	Sex	Diagnosis	Surgical procedure	Type of anesthesia	Witnessed/ assisted

List of drugs used in operation theatre

Sl. No.	Name of the drug	Indication	Action	Dosage	Side effects

List of nurses responsibilities in the operation theatre

1. _____
2. _____
3. _____
4. _____
5. _____
6. _____
7. _____
8. _____
9. _____
10. _____

Preoperative care: [What has been performed/done?]

_____
_____
_____
_____
_____
_____

Postoperative care: [What has been performed/done?]

_____

_____

_____

_____

_____

References

_____

_____

_____

_____

_____

Annexure I
Sample of Nursing Care Plan

HISTORY TAKING

I. Identification data:

a.	Name	:	Ramappa Kamate
b.	Address	:	A/p Mallapur PG Ta: Gokak Dist: Belgaum
c.	Age	:	75 yrs
d.	Sex	:	Male
e.	Marital status	:	Married
f.	Education	:	Illiterate
g.	Occupation	:	Former
h.	Income	:	50,000/-
i.	Religion	:	Hindu
j.	IP No.	:	12320
k.	Diagnosis	:	Bronchitis
l.	Date of admission	:	20/04/2014

II. Presenting chief complaints: [Write down the client's problem as per their verbatim in chronological order.]

- Cough with sputum since one week
- Fever and chills since 5 days
- Chest pain since 5 days
- Loss of appetite since yesterday

III. History of present illness: [Explain the client's problem with aggravating factors, relieving factor, precipitating factors, its characteristics, intensity, etc.]

Low grade fever is followed by chills then sweating which is associated with cough and sputum since last five days cough is reduced in the sitting position and relieved after sputum expelled out.

IV. Past history of illness: [Explain the past medical, surgical history with its treatment, etc.] there is no history of DM/HTN/cardiac illness, etc. and he has been hospitalized in the local clinic for one day before arriving in this hospital.

V. Family history: [Family structure/family health history/social support system, etc.]

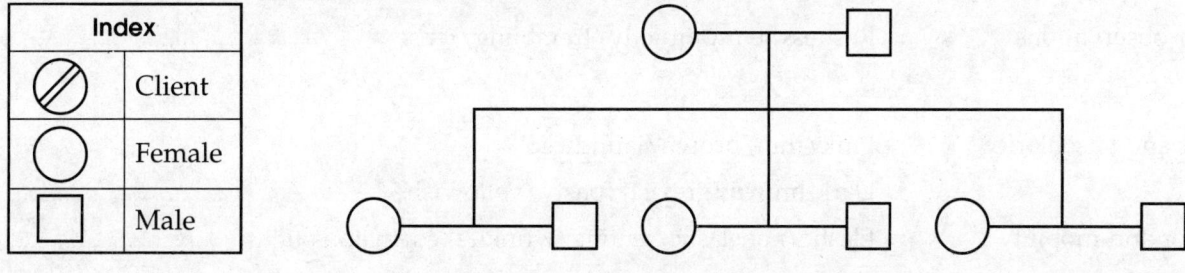

Index	
⊘	Client
◯	Female
☐	Male

Sl. No.	Name of the family members	Relationship with patient	Age/sex	Educational status	Occupational status	Marital status	Health status
1.	Mallappa	HOF	75/M	Illiterate	Former	Married	Unhealthy
2.	Devaki	Wife	68/F	Illiterate	House wife	Married	Healthy
3.	Rajeev	Son	48/M	10th	Former	Married	Healthy
4.	Parvati	Daughter-in-law	39/F	8th	House wife	Married	Healthy
5.	Raghu	Son	45/M	12th	Former	Married	Healthy
6.	Laxmidevi	Daughter-in-law	34/F	8th	Hosue wife	Married	Healthy
7.	Rohit	Grandson	10/M	4th	Student	Unmarried	Healthy
8.	Rohini	Granddaughter	8/F	2nd	Student	Unmarried	Healthy
9.							
10.							

VI. Personal history: [Bowel, bladder, sleep, diet, habit, etc.]
- Bowel : Regular
- Bladder : Regular
- Sleep : Disturbed
- Diet : Non veg
- Habit : Alcoholic and tobacco

PHYSICAL EXAMINATION

Note: Students are instructed to follow the descriptive terminologies for documentation of physical examination and write suitable terms in the space given:

General Appearance

Level of consciousness : Conscious/unconscious/semiconscious/coma ....

Activity : Active/dull/lethargic ....

Body built : Mild/moderate/thin/obese/emaciated/flabby ....

Height : ....

Weight : ....

General grooming : Clean/combed/make-up ....

Body language : Eye contact/no eye contact/arms folded over chest ....

Other observations : Restless/lying quietly/trembling/tense ....

Skin

Color and vascularity : Pink/thin/brown/jaundiced
Dark brown/greyish/pasty/yellowish ....

Turgor and mobility : Elastic/nonelastic/tenting/wrinkles/edematous tight ....

Temperature and moisture	:	Cold/cool/warm/hot/feverish/sweating Moisty/dry/clammy/oily/diaphoresis.	....
Texture	:	Smooth/rough/fine/thick/scaly/puffy	....
Nails	:	Clean manicured/smooth/rough/yellowish/ paronychia.	....
		Dry/hard/brittle/splitting/cracking/angle of nail bed/clubbing/curved/flat/thick.	....
Body hair growth	:	Color/thick/thin/fine/coarse/hirsutism	....
Skin integrity	:	Intact/not intact/birth marks/scars/moles	....
Lesions	:	Lesions/fissures/abrasion/cysts/wheals/erythema/ pimples/black heads/scaly/laceration/ulcers	....

Head

Shape	:	Round/oval/square/pointed/normocephalic	....
Face	:	Oval/heart shaped/pear/long square symmetrical/ round/thin/high-cheeked bone	....
Sensation	:	Trigeminal cranial nerve/facial cranial nerve	....
Hair	:	Color and growth/fine/thin/alopecia	....
Condition of the scalp	:	Clean/scaly/dandruff/rashes/sores	....
Facial puffiness	:	Present/absent	....

Eyes

Eyebrows	:	Color/shape alignment/straight/curve/thick/thin	....
Eyelashes	:	Long/short/curve/artificial	....
Eyelids	:	Dark/swollen/inflamed/stye/ptosis/entropion/ ectropion/xanthomas/open and closed simultaneously	....
Shape and appearance	:	Almond/rounded/prominent/nystagmus/ exophthalmus/sunken/bright/tearing/discharge	....
Sclera	:	White/cream/yellowish/infected/jaundiced	....
Conjunctiva	:	Pale pink/pink/red/inflamed/swelling	....
Iris	:	Color/shape/round/flat	....
Cornea	:	Clear/milky/opaque/cloudy	....
Pupils	:	Occulomotor cranial nerve/size and shape/equality/ symmetrical/reaction to light/dilated/constricted/ unequal/fixed	....
Visual field	:	Intact/not intact	....
Vision	:	Reads/reports	....
Use of glasses	:	Glasses/contact lenses/prosthesis	....

Ears

Pinnae : Size and shape/small or large in proportion to face/ large or small lobes/symmetrical/skin intact/ redness/swelling ....

Level in relation to eyes : Top of the pinnae level with outer canthus of the eyes ....

Canal : Clean/discharge/redness/foreign object ....

Cilia : Present/absent ....

Cerumen : Present/absent/color consistency ....

Tympanic membrane : Color/peary white/red inflamed/cone of light/ land mark/bubbles/fluid level ....

Hearing (audition) : Vestibulocochlear nerve/hearing present or absent both side ....

Tuning fork test : Listen/not listen ....

Weber test : Lateralizes equally to left/right side ....

Rinne test : Air conduction/bone conduction 2 : 1 ....

Hearing aid : Yes/no, right/left ....

Nose and Sinuses

Size and shape : Long/short/small/large/flat/broad/thick/ thin/symmetrical/pointed/flaring of nostrils ....

Nasal septum : Midline/deviated to right or left/perforated ....

Nasal mucosa and turbinate : Pink/pale/bluish/red/dry/moist/discharge/cilia/ epistaxis/polyps ....

Patency of nares : Right patent/partial obstruction ....

Olfactory : Identification of sense of smell/odor ....

Sinuses : Tender/nontender/transillumination ....

Mouth and Pharynx

Lips : Pink/red/pale/cyanotic ....

Teeth : White/yellowish/grayish/spotted/stained/ irregular/broken/loose teeth ....

Dental caries and fillings : Number and location ....

Dental hygiene : Clean/not clean ....

Breath odor : Sweet/odorless/halitosis/foul/musty/acetone/ alcohol/odor of drug ....

Gums : Pink/firm/swollen/bleeding/gingivitis/irritated/ moist/dry/ulcerated ....

Facial and glossopharyngeal nerve : Identifies taste ....

Tongue	:	Thick/thin/pink/pale/bluish/glossitis/ ulcer/coated	....
Hypoglossal	:	Tongue movement/symmetry/lateral/ fasciculation	....
Mucosa	:	Color/leukoplakia/dry/moist/intact/not intact	....
Palate	:	Moist/dry/color	....
Uvula	:	Color/midline	....
Pharynx	:	Color/petechiae/infected/dysphagia	....
Tonsils	:	Present/absent/crypt	....
Temporomandibular joint	:	Fully mobile symmetry/tenderness/crepitus	....

Neck

Appearance	:	Long/short/thick/thin/masses/size and shape/ symmetry	....
Thyroid	:	Palpable/nodules/tender	
Trachea	:	Midline/deviated to right/left	....
Lymph nodes	:	Palpation of lymph nodes (lymphadenopathy) hard/firm	....

Thorax and Lungs

Respiratory rate/rhythm	:	Tachypnea/bradypnea/orthopnea/stertorous/ regular/irregular/gasping/deep/shallow	....
Thoracic cage shape	:	Barrel/pigeon/scoliosis/kyphosis/normal	....
Configuration	:	Pectus excavation/pectus carinatum/normal	....
Skin color and condition	:	Normal/cyanosis/pallor	....
Chest examination	:	Symmetric/asymmetric	....
Posterior thorax	:	Tenderness/masses/respiratory excursion/ symmetric/asymmetric/no respiratory movement on left or right side/crepitus/ resonance/dull/emphysema	....
Percussion of lung field	:	Clear/not clear	....
Diaphragmatic exertion	:	Dull/normal	....
Lung auscultation	:	Vascular/bronchovascular/bronchial/whispered/ rales/rhonchi/crackles/rub	....
Breath sound	:	Vascular/bronchovascular	....
Respiratory pattern	:	Normal/abnormal	....

Breast and Axillae

| Male breasts | : | Lumps/swelling/gynecomastia | .... |
| Female breasts | : | Symmetry/pain discharge/trauma/abnormalities/ surgeries | .... |

| Nipples | : | Symmetrical/circular/inverted/everted/pale/ brown/discharge | .... |
| Axillae | : | Shaved/unshaved/odor/lump masses | .... |

Cardiovascular Examination

Heart	:	Precardial bulge/abnormal palpitation/point of maximal impulse (PMI)/thrills/S1, S2, S3, S4/ clicks/snap/rub/gallop	....
Heart sound	:	S1, S2 heard/abnormalities	....
Murmurs	:	Systolic/diastolic/holosystolic/harsh/soft/ blowing/rumbling/high, medium, low pitch	....
Carotid pulse	:	Volume/rhythm	....
Apical pulse	:	Tachycardia/bradycardia/pounding forceful, weak/regular/irregular	....
Peripheral pulses	:	Volume/rhythm/symmetry	....
Blood pressure/pulse rate	:		....

Abdominal Examination

Contour	:	Irregular/protruding/enlarged/distended/scaphoid/ concave/sunken/firm/flat/flaccid	....
Skin	:	Intact/shiny/smooth scar/lesion/striae/umbilicus	....
Bowel sounds	:	Present/absent/hyperactive/high-pitched tickling/ gurgles	....
On percussion	:	Tympanic/dull/flat/ascites/fluid collection	....
Palpation	:	Splenomegaly/hepatomegaly/organomegaly/aortic pulse/tenderness/bulges/hernias/lymph nodes	....

Musculoskeletal Examination

Back	:	Shoulder level alignment/lordosis/scoliosis/ kyphosis	....
Vertebral column alignment	:	Straight/lordosis/scoliosis/kyphosis/ankylosis	....
Range of motion	:	Full/limited/fixed (all joints)	....
Extremities	:	Color/symmetry/variation/temperature/muscle tone/tomor	....
Lower extremities	:	Symmetry/variation/prosthesis/varicose vein	....

Genitourinary and Rectum

| Rectum | : | Hemorrhoids/fissures/inflammation/lesion/ swelling/rectocele | .... |

Female genitalia   : Pubic hair/lesions/nodules/swelling/pigmentations/
                           dry/moist/discharge/odor/uterine prolapse/rashes   ....

Male genitalia   : Pubic hair/color/circumcision/phimosis/hydrocele/
                           epispodiasis/hypospadiasis/rash/discharge/edema/
                           scrotal sac rugated/atrophy   ....

Neurological Examination

Describes tics, twitches,
paresthesias   :   ....

Gait   : Balanced/shuffling/unsteady/ataxic/parkinsonism/
                           scissor/spastic   ....

Cranial nerves   : Accessory nerve   ....

Reflexes   : Present/absent   ....

Co-ordination   : Report as to test done   ....

Mental Status Examination

Level of alertness   : Alert/stuperous/semiconscious   ....

Orientation   : Time/place/person   ....

Memory   : Recent memory/long-term memory   ....

Language and speech   : Language/speech/slow/rapid/slurred/difficulty in
                           forming words aphasia   ....

Responsiveness   : Responds to verbal stimuli—slow/rapid   ....

Knowledge test   :   ....

Thinking   :   ....

Judgment   :   ....

Insight   :   ....

Investigation

Sl. No.	Name of investigation	Client's value	Normal value	Remarks
1.	Hemoglobin	12 gm%	12–14 gm%	Normal
2.	Total leukocyte count	3500	4000–11000	Leukocytopenia
3.	Neutrophils	72%	65–75%	Normal
4.	Lymphocyte	25%	20–25%	Normal
5.	Monocyte	0%	0–2%	Normal
6.	Basophils	1%	0–2%	Normal
7.	Eosinophil	2%	2–4%	Normal
8.	ESR	9–20 after 1 hour	30	Abnormal
9.	HIV	–ve	–ve	Normal
10.	Moutoux test	–ve	–ve	Normal

Treatment/Medications

Sl. No.	Name of drug	Dosage	Frequency	Class of drug
1.	Inj Hiceff	1 gm	BID	Cephalosporin anti-microbial
2.	Inj Rantac	1 amp	BID	H_2 receptor
3.	Inj Dolonex	1 amp	BID	NSAID
4.	Syp Brutus	2 tsp	TID	Expectorant
5.				
6.				
7.				
8.				
9.				
10.				

Nursing diagnosis: List down the nursing diagnosis based on needs and problems of the client with priority [Maslow's hierarchy].

- Ineffective airway clearance related to sputum production
- Chest pain related to inflammatory process
- Impaired body temperature more than normal related to infection
- Altered sleep pattern related to cough
- Anxiety related to hospitalization
- Activity intolerance related to fatigue and decreased nutritional status.

Care plan: Prepare the plan of care with priority [at least 5 need-based care to be given].

Assessment	Diagnosis	Objectives	Intervention	Evaluation
Subjective data: Patient complaining of cough and sputum **Objective data:** By observing amount of sputum secretion and breathing pattern	Ineffective airway clearance related to sputum production	Airway will be cleared	Assess the severity of cough and type of sputum. Suctioning to be done. Perform chest physiotherapy. Assess the breathing pattern. Give medication as per doctor's advice	Airway cleared
Subjective data: Patient complaining of chest pain **Objective data:** By observing patients expressions	Chest pain related to inflammatory process	Chest pain will be relieved	Assess the chest pain. Provide psychological support. Give medication as per doctor's advice	Chest pain relieved

(Contd.)

Assessment	Diagnosis	Objectives	Intervention	Evaluation
Subjective data: Patient complaining of fever **Objective data:** By recording body temperature of patient	Impaired body temperature more than normal related to infection	Body temperature will be reduced	Assess the body temperature every 2 hourly. Give cross ventilation. Give cold compress. Give plenty of oral fluids. Give antipyretics as per doctor's advice	Body temperature reduced to normal
Subjective data: Patient complaining of sleeplessness **Objective data:** Patient feels drowsiness	Altered sleep pattern related to cough	Sleeping pattern will be normal	Assess the sleeping pattern. Provide comfort devices. Provide psychological support. Provide calm and quiet environment for complete rest	Sleeping pattern becomes normal
Subjective data: Patient complaining of anxiety about various procedures **Objective data:** By verbalization of patient about procedures done on the patients	Anxiety related to hospitalization	Anxiety will be relieved	Assess the condition of the patient. Be with the patient always. Give psychological support. Explain every procedure done on the patient to alleviate anxiety	Anxiety relieved

Health education: List down the health education topics, prepare AV aids and impart the education.

- Educate the patient and family about chest physiotherapy.
- Educate them about postural drainage.
- Encourage the patient for active exercises
- Advice about nutritional diet.
- Educate about personal hygiene.
- Advice about regular follow-up and medication.

Final impression and suspected illness/disease [states the problems or nursing diagnosis]

_____

_____

_____

_____

_____

_____

Annexure II
Sample of Nursing Care Study/Presentation

VII. Identification data:

a.	Name	: Ramappa Kamate
b.	Address	: A/p Mallapur PG Ta: Gokak Dist: Belgaum
c.	Age	: 75 yrs
d.	Sex	: Male
e.	Marital status	: Married
f.	Education	: Illiterate
g.	Occupation	: Former
h.	Income	: 50,000/-
i.	Religion	: Hindu
j.	IP No.	: 12320
k.	Diagnosis	: Bronchitis
l.	Date of admission	: 20/04/2014

VIII. Reason for selection of the study: [Give brief description.]

I have selected this case for nursing case/presentation as a partial fulfilment of requirement that this condition is in the curriculum and this client was conscious and co-operative while interview.

IX. Presenting chief complaints: [Write down the client's problem as per their verbatim in chronological order.]

- Cough with sputum since one week
- Fever and chills since 5 days
- Chest pain since 5 days
- Loss of appetite since yesterday

X. History of present illness: [Explain the client's problem with aggravating factors, relieving factor, precipitating factors, its characteristics, intensity, etc.]

Low grade fever is followed by chills then sweating which is associated with cough and sputum since last five days cough is reduced in the sitting position and relieved after sputum expelled out.

XI. Past history of illness: [Explain the past medical, surgical history with its treatment, etc.] there is no history of DM/HTN/cardiac illness, etc. and he has been hospitalized in the local clinic for one day before arriving in this hospital.

XII. Family history: [Family structure/family health history/social support system, etc.]

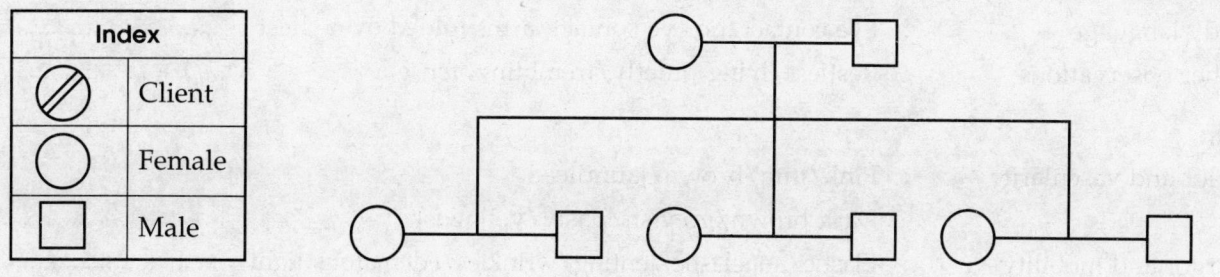

Index	
⊘	Client
◯	Female
☐	Male

Sl. No.	Name of the family members	Relationship with patient	Age/sex	Educational status	Occupational status	Marital status	Health status
1.	Mallappa	HOF	75/M	Illiterate	Former	Married	Unhealthy
2.	Devaki	Wife	68/F	Illiterate	House wife	Married	Healthy
3.	Rajeev	Son	48/M	10th	Former	Married	Healthy
4.	Parvati	Daughter-in-law	39/F	8th	House wife	Married	Healthy
5.	Raghu	Son	45/M	12th	Former	Married	Healthy
6.	Laxmidevi	Daughter-in-law	34/F	8th	Hosue wife	Married	Healthy
7.	Rohit	Grandson	10/M	4th	Student	Unmarried	Healthy
8.	Rohini	Granddaughter	8/F	2nd	Student	Unmarried	Healthy
9.							
10.							

XIII. Personal history: [Bowel, bladder, sleep, diet, habit, etc.]

- Bowel   : Regular
- Bladder   : Regular
- Sleep   : Disturbed
- Diet   : Non veg
- Habit   : Alcoholic and tobacco

PHYSICAL EXAMINATION

Note: Students are instructed to follow the descriptive terminologies for documentation of physical examination and write suitable terms in the space given:

General Appearance

Level of consciousness	:	Conscious/unconscious/semiconscious/coma	....
Activity	:	Active/dull/lethargic	....
Body built	:	Mild/moderate/thin/obese/emaciated/flabby	....
Height	:		....
Weight	:		....
General grooming	:	Clean/combed/make-up	....

Body language : Eye contact/no eye contact/arms folded over chest ....

Other observations : Restless/lying quietly/trembling/tense ....

Skin

Color and vascularity : Pink/thin/brown/jaundiced

Dark brown/greyish/pasty/yellowish ....

Turgor and mobility : Elastic/nonelastic/tenting/wrinkles/edematous tight ....

Temperature and moisture : Cold/cool/warm/hot/feverish/sweating

Moisty/dry/clammy/oily/diaphoresis ....

Texture : Smooth/rough/fine/thick/scaly/puffy ....

Nails : Clean manicured/smooth/rough/yellowish/

paronychia ....

Dry/hard/brittle/splitting/cracking/angle of nail

bed/clubbing/curved/flat/thick. ....

Body hair growth : Color/thick/thin/fine/coarse/hirsutism ....

Skin integrity : Intact/not intact/birth marks/scars/moles ....

Lesions : Lesions/fissures/abrasion/cysts/wheals/erythema/

pimples/black heads/scaly/laceration/ulcers ....

Head

Shape : Round/oval/square/pointed/normocephalic ....

Face : Oval/heart shaped/pear/long square symmetrical/

round/thin/high-cheeked bone ....

Sensation : Trigeminal cranial nerve/facial cranial nerve ....

Hair : Color and growth/fine/thin/alopecia ....

Condition of the scalp : Clean/scaly/dandruff/rashes/sores ....

Facial puffiness : Present/absent ....

Eyes

Eyebrows : Color/shape alignment/straight/curve/thick/thin ....

Eyelashes : Long/short/curve/artificial ....

Eyelids : Dark/swollen/inflamed/stye/ptosis/entropion/

ectropion/xanthomas/open and closed

simultaneously ....

Shape and appearance : Almond/rounded/prominent/nystagmus/

exophthalmus/sunken/bright/tearing/discharge ....

Sclera : White/cream/yellowish/infected/jaundiced ....

Conjunctiva : Pale pink/pink/red/inflamed/swelling ....

Iris : Color/shape/round/flat ....

Cornea : Clear/milky/opaque/cloudy ....

Pupils	:	Occulomotor cranial nerve/size and shape/equality/ symmetrical/reaction to light/dilated/constricted/ unequal/fixed ....
Visual field	:	Intact/not intact ....
Vision	:	Reads/reports ....
Use of glasses	:	Glasses/contact lenses/prosthesis ....

Ears

Pinnae	:	Size and shape/small or large in proportion to face/ large or small lobes/symmetrical/skin intact/ redness/swelling ....
Level in relation to eyes	:	Top of the pinnae level with outer canthus of the eyes ....
Canal	:	Clean/discharge/redness/foreign object ....
Cilia	:	Present/absent ....
Cerumen	:	Present/absent/color consistency ....
Tympanic membrane	:	Color/peary white/red inflamed/cone of light/ landmark/bubbles/fluid level ....
Hearing (audition)	:	Vestibulocochlear nerve/hearing present or absent both side ....
Tuning fork test	:	Listen/not listen ....
Weber test	:	Lateralizes equally to left/right side ....
Rinne test	:	Air conduction/bone conduction 2 : 1 ....
Hearing aid	:	Yes/no, right/left ....

Nose and Sinuses

Size and shape	:	Long/short/small/large/flat/broad/thick/ thin/symmetrical/pointed/flaring of nostrils ....
Nasal septum	:	Midline/deviated to right or left/perforated ....
Nasal mucosa and turbinate	:	Pink/pale/bluish/red/dry/moist/discharge/cilia/ epistaxis/polyps ....
Patency of nares	:	Right patent/partial obstruction ....
Olfactory	:	Identification of sense of smell/odor ....
Sinuses	:	Tender/nontender/transillumination ....

Mouth and Pharynx

Lips	:	Pink/red/pale/cyanotic ....
Teeth	:	White/yellowish/grayish/spotted/stained/ irregular/broken/loose teeth ....
Dental caries and fillings	:	Number and location ....
Dental hygiene	:	Clean/not clean ....

Breath odor	: Sweet/odorless/halitosis/foul/musty/acetone/ alcohol/odor of drug	....
Gums	: Pink/firm/swollen/bleeding/gingivitis/irritated/ moist/dry/ulcerated	....
Facial and glossopharyngeal nerve	: Identifies taste	....
Tongue	: Thick/thin/pink/pale/bluish/glossitis/ ulcer/coated	....
Hypoglossal	: Tongue movement/symmetry/lateral/ fasciculation	....
Mucosa	: Color/leukoplakia/dry/moist/intact/not intact	....
Palate	: Moist/dry/color	....
Uvula	: Color/midline	....
Pharynx	: Color/patechiae/infected/dysphagia	....
Tonsils	: Present/absent/crypt	....
Temporomandibular joint	: Fully mobile symmetry/tenderness/crepitus	....

Neck

Appearance	: Long/short/thick/thin/masses/size and shape/ symmetry	....
Thyroid	: Palpable/nodules/tender	....
Trachea	: Midline/deviated to right/left	....
Lymph nodes	: Palpation of lymph nodes (lymphadenopathy) hard/firm	....

Thorax and Lungs

Respiratory rate/rhythm	: Tachypnea/Bradypnea/orthopnea/stertorous/ regular/irregular/gasping/deep/shallow	....
Thoracic cage shape	: Barrel/pigeon/scoliosis/kyphosis/normal	....
Configuration	: Pectus excavation/pectus carinatum/normal	....
Skin color and condition	: Normal/cyanosis/pallor	....
Chest examination	: Symmetric/asymmetric	....
Posterior thorax	: Tenderness/masses/respiratory excursion/ symmetric/asymmetric/no respiratory movement on left or right side/crepitus/ resonance/dull/emphysema	....
Percussion of lung field	: Clear/not clear	....
Diaphragmatic exertion	: Dull/normal	....
Lung auscultation	: Vascular/bronchovascular/bronchial/whispered/ rales/rhonchi/crackles/rub	....

| Breath sound | : | Vascular/bronchovascular | .... |
| Respiratory pattern | : | Normal/abnormal | .... |

Breast and Axillae

Male breasts	:	Lumps/swelling/gynecomastia	
Female breasts	:	Symmetry/pain discharge/trauma/abnormalities/ surgeries	
			....
Nipples	:	Symmetrical/circular/inverted/eeverted/pale/ brown/discharge	
			....
Axillae	:	Shaved/unshaved/odor/lump masses	....

Cardiovascular Examination

Heart	:	Precardial bulge/abnormal palpitation/point of maximal impulse (PMI)/thrills/S1, S2, S3, S4/ clicks/snap/rub/gallop	
Heart sound	:	S1, S2 heard/abnormalities	
Murmurs	:	Systolic/diastolic/holosystolic/harsh/soft/ blowing/rumbling/high, medium, low pitched	
			....
Carotid pulse	:	Volume/rhythm	....
Apical pulse	:	Tachycardia/bradycardia/pounding forceful, weak/regular/irregular	
			....
Peripheral pulses	:	Volume/rhythm/symmetry	....
Blood pressure/pulse rate	:		

Abdominal Examination

Contour	:	Irregular/protruding/enlarged/distended/scaphoid/ concave/sunken/firm/flat/flaccid	
Skin	:	Intact/shiny/smooth scar/lesion/striae/umbilicus	....
Bowel sounds	:	Present/absent/hyperactive/high-pitched tickling/ gurgles	
			....
On percussion	:	Tympanic/dull/flat/ascites/fluid collection	....
Palpation	:	Splenomegaly/hepatomegaly/organomegaly/aortic pulse/tenderness/bulges/hernias/lymph nodes	
			....

Musculoskeletal Examination

Back	:	Shoulder level alignment/lordosis/scoliosis/ kyphosis	
			....
Vertebral column alignment	:	Straight/lordosis/scoliosis/kyphosis/ankylosis	....
Range of motion	:	Full/limited/fixed (all joints)	

| Extremities | : | Color/symmetry/variation/temperature/muscle tone/tomor | .... |
| Lower extremities | : | Symmetry/variation/prosthesis/varicose vein | .... |

Genitourinary and Rectum

Rectum	:	Hemorrhoids/fissures/inflammation/lesion/ swelling/rectocele	....
Female genitalia	:	Pubic hair/lesions/nodules/swelling/ pigmentations/dry/moist/discharge/odor/ uterine prolapse/rashes	....
Male genitalia	:	Pubic hair/color/circumcision/phimosis/hydrocele/ epispadiasis/hypospodiasis/rash/discharge/edema/ scrotal sac rugated/atrophy	....

Neurological Examination

Describes tics, twitches, paresthesias	:		....
Gait	:	Balanced/shuffling/unsteady/ataxic/parkinsonism/ scissor/spastic	....
Cranial nerves	:	Accessory nerve	....
Reflexes	:	Present/absent	....
Co-ordination	:	Report as to test done	....

Mental Status Examination

Level of alertness	:	Alert/stuperous/semiconscious	....
Orientation	:	Time/place/person	....
Memory	:	Recent memory/long-term memory	....
Language and speech	:	Language/speech/slow/rapid/slurred/difficulty in forming words aphasia	....
Responsiveness	:	Responds to verbal stimuli—slow/rapid	....
Knowledge test	:		....
Thinking	:		....
Judgment	:		....
Insight	:		....

DESCRIPTION OF PRESENT DISEASE

Introduction

Bronchitis is common upper respiratory tract infection among all the age group of people it requires keen observation and identification of cause of the illness and removal of victim from the environment provide comprehensive nursing care to the patient with bronchitis.

Definition

Bronchitis is an inflammation of the bronchi and bronchiole of the lungs.

Related Anatomy and Physiology [give brief note]

The bronchi are composed of the same tissues as the trachea. They are lined with ciliated columnar epithelium. The bronchi progressively subdivided into bronchioles, alveolar duct and finally alveoli.

Functions

1. Control of airway
2. Warning and humidifying
3. Cough reflex
4. Removal of dust and foreign particles by cough and sputum production

Etiology/risk factors [mention present causes, possible causes and risk factors and compare with book picture].

Etiology and risk factors	Book picture
Inflamed airway and irritated with increased mucus production.	Primary viral etiology but may also arise from bacterial agents. Inflamed airway and irritated with increased mucus production.

Pathophysiology: [Mention present pathophysiology of the patient and compared with book picture.]

In many cases smoke or other environmental pollutants irritate the airway

↓

This cause hypersecretion of due to inflammation

↓

Constant irritation causes mucus secretion from the goblet cells

↓

This leads to reduction in the cilliary functions and more production of the mucus

↓

Causes thickening of the bronchial wall and narrowing of the bronchi and bronchioles

↓

This leads to altered functions in the alveolar macrophage functions

↓

In wide range of the viral, bacterial, mycoplasmal infections can produce acute episode of the bronchitis

Clinical Manifestations

Signs and symptoms of the patient	Book picture
Fever with chills	Dyspnea, fever, tachypnea
Cough with sputum	Productive cough to removal the sputum
Chest pain	Pleuritic chest pain
Loss of sleep and weakness	Diffuse bronchi
Breathlessness	Irritation of the mucosa

Investigation

Sl. No.	Name of investigation	Client's value	Normal value	Remarks
1.	Hemoglobin	12 gm%	12–14 gm%	Normal
2.	Total leukocyte count	3500	4000–11000	Leukocytopenia
3.	Neutrophils	72%	65–75%	Normal
4.	Lymphocyte	25%	20–25%	Normal
5.	Monocyte	0%	0–2%	Normal
6.	Basophils	1%	0–2%	Normal
7.	Eosinophil	2%	2–4%	Normal
8.	ESR	9–20 after 1 hour	30	Abnormal
9.	HIV	–ve	–ve	Normal
10.	Moutoux test	–ve	–ve	Normal

Treatment/Medications

Sl. No.	Name of drug	Dosage	Route	Frequency	Side effects	Nurses responsibilities
1.	Inj Hiceff	1 gm	IV	BID		
2.	Inj Rantac	1 amp	IV	BID		
3.	Inj Dolonex	1 amp	IM	BID		
4.	Syp Brutus	2 tsp	Oral	BID		
5.						

Nursing diagnosis: List down the nursing diagnosis based on needs and problems of the client with priority [Maslow's hierarchy].

- Ineffective airway clearance related to sputum production.
- Chest pain related to inflammatory process.
- Impaired body temperature more than normal related to infection.
- Altered sleep pattern related to cough.
- Anxiety related to hospitalization.
- Activity intolerance related to fatigue and decreased nutritional status.

Care plan: Prepare the plan of care with priority [at least 5 need-based care to be given].

Assessment	Diagnosis	Objectives	Intervention	Evaluation
Subjective data: Patient complaining of cough and sputum **Objective data:** By observing amount of sputum secretion and breathing pattern	Ineffective airway clearance related to sputum production	Airway will be cleared	Assess the severity of cough and type of sputum. Suctioning to be done. Perform chest physiotherapy. Assess the breathing pattern. Give medication as per doctor's advice	Airway cleared
Subjective data: Patient complaining of chest pain **Objective data:** By observing patients expressions	Chest pain related to inflammatory process	Chest pain will be relieved	Assess the chest pain. Provide psychological support. Give medication as per doctor's advice	Chest pain relieved
Subjective data: Patient complaining of fever **Objective data:** By recording body temperature of patient	Impaired body temperature more than normal related to infection	Body temperature will be reduced.	Assess the body temperature every 2 hourly. Give cross ventilation. Give cold compress. Give plenty of oral fluids. Give antipyretics as per doctor's advice	Body temperature reduced to normal
Subjective data: Patient complaining of sleeplessness **Objective data:** Patient feels drowsiness	Altered sleep pattern related to cough	Sleeping pattern will be normal	Assess the sleeping pattern. Provide comfort devices. Provide psychological support. Provide calm and quiet environment for complete rest	Sleeping pattern becomes normal
Subjective data: Patient complaining of anxiety about various procedures **Objective data:** By verbalization of patient about procedures done on the patients	Anxiety related to hospitalization	Anxiety will be relieved	Assess the condition of the patient. Be with the patient always. Give psychological support. Explain every procedure done on the patient to alleviate anxiety	Anxiety relieved

Health education: List down the health education topics, prepare AV aids and impart the education.

- Educate the patient and family about chest physiotherapy.
- Educate them about postural drainage.
- Encourage the patient for active exercises
- Advice about nutritional diet.
- Educate about personal hygiene.
- Advice about regular follow-up and medication.

Final impression and suspected illness/disease [states the problems or nursing diagnosis]

_____

_____

_____

_____

_____

_____

_____

Summary and Conclusion

By studying this disease condition I came to know in detail about bronchitis and providing comprehensive care to the patient with bronchitis.

Bibliography

1. Lippincot Williams and Wilkins textbook of medical surgical nursing. 8th edition, pp. 1066–1080.
2. Joyce M. Black textbook of medical surgical nursing. 7th edition, pp. 778–790.
3.
4.
5.
6.

Annexure III
Sample of Bedside Procedure

XIV. Identification data:

a.	Name	: Ramappa Kamate
b.	Address	: A/p Mallapur PG Ta: Gokak Dist: Belgaum
c.	Age	: 75 yrs
d.	Sex	: Male
e.	Marital status	: Married
f.	Education	: Illiterate
g.	Occupation	: Former
h.	Income	: 50,000/-
i.	Religion	: Hindu
j.	IP No.	: 12320
k.	Diagnosis	: Bronchitis
l.	Date of admission	: 20/04/2014

Definition

Bronchitis is an inflammation of the bronchi and bronchiole of the lungs.

Nursing assessment: Mention the key points of subjective and objective data

- Cough with sputum since one week
- Fever and chills since 5 days
- Chest pain since 5 days
- Loss of appetite since yesterday
- On observation body temperature is 99°F
- Pulse rate 100/min
- RR is 20/min
- Restlessness.

Nursing diagnosis: List of problems based on priority [Maslow's hierarchy]

- Ineffective airway clearance related to sputum production
- Chest pain related to inflammatory process
- Impaired body temperature more than normal related to infection

173

- Altered sleep pattern related to cough
- Anxiety related to hospitalization
- Activity intolerance related to fatigue and decreased nutritional status.

Planning: State the objectives of the care

1. To provide comfortable position by providing comfort devices.

2. To clear the airway by postural drainage and chest physiotherapy.

3. To maintain personal hygiene.

4. To maintain nutritional status.

Intervention: State the interventions to be performed

1. Provide comfort devices

2. Maintain clear airway by postural drainage and chest physiotherapy

3. Maintain personal hygiene

4. Provide nutritious diet.

Nursing procedure: Related to client condition

- **Name of the procedure: Nail care**
- **Definition of the procedure:**
  - Nail care is the simplest procedure to give care to the client who are unable to self-care of their nail.
- **Purpose of the procedure:**
  - To keep the nail clean and dry.
  - To teach the patient and family about nail care.
  - To trim the nail short to prevent injuries to the tissues.
  - To prevent accumulation of dirt and microorganism underneath the nail.
  - To prevent odor
  - To promote circulation to the nail buds
  - To prevent abnormal appearance

Articles required for procedure:
Preparation of the client:

1. Mackintosh and towel to protect linen from soiling

2. Small bowl with warm water disinfectant solution for soaking the nail

3. Nail cutter to trim the nails

4. Kidney tray or paper bag to receive wastages

5. Pads to receive nail cut particles.

6. A bowl containing dry swab for drying the nails.

Steps of the procedures with rationale

Sl. No.	Steps of the procedure	Rationale
	Explain the procedure to patient	To gain confidence and co-operation of patient
	Remove watch and wash the hands	To minimize cross infection
	Arrange all the articles beside the bed	To prevent energy while doing procedure
	Place the patient in sitting position and inspect the nails of finger and toes	
	Spread the mackintosh and towel	To prevent soiling of linen
	Soak the nails of finger and toes	To prevent cracking of nails and injury to the tissues of nail buds
	Trim the nails with nail cutter	
	File the nails after cutting the nails	To smoothen the nails
	Dry the nails with dry swabs	

Care of the client after procedure:

Replace all the articles to utility rooms after cleaning of articles.

Care of the articles/area:

Observe for the circulation of the nail buds and maintain cleanliness of fingers and toe nails.

Coments

_____

_____

_____

_____

Health Teaching

Give health education to the patient and family about care of the finger and toe nails for prevention of the cross infections and accumulation of dirt and microorganisms in the nail buds.

Explain the procedure of nail care to them.

Annexure IV
Sample of Drug Study

Trade name	:	Mezole, Flagyl
Generic name	:	Metronidazole
Drug group	:	Anti-amoebic drug
Mode of action	:	The exact mechanism of action of the drug is unknown or not clear but probable mechanism is drug enters into the cytoplasm. In the cytoplasm it produces some toxic chemicals, these toxic chemicals may damage the DNA and other critical biomolecules due to the damage of the DNA, amoeba may die so it has a amoebicidal action.
Indication of drug	:	Giardiasis, trichomonas, vaginitis, anaerobic bacterial infections, pseudomembranous enterocolitis, ulcerative gingivitis, *H. pylori* gastritis and peptic ulcer, gynecological infections.
Dosage	:	Adult: 750 mg thrice daily for 5–10 days Children: 30–50 mg/kg /day for 5–10 days in three divided doses
Route of administration	:	Oral and intravenous infusion
Side effects	:	Anorexia, nausea, vomiting, dizziness, abdominal cramps, headache, glossitis, dryness of mouth, rashes and transient neutropenia.
Contraindication	:	Neurological disease, blood dyscrasias, seizures and hepatic failure.
Nurses responsibilities	:	Monitor liver function test. Observe for edema In case of vaginal infections every partner with asymptomatic is given metronidazole prophylactically.

References

1. Drug index, CIMS, MIMS latest editions.
2. Mosby's nurses drug guide.

Annexure V
Sample of Health Talk

Name of student–teacher : ABC

Year : Individual/family/community
Group

Subject : Personal hygiene

Topic : Oral hygiene

Group and size : Individual or group

Method of teaching : Lecturer cum discussion

AV aids : Flash card/poster/chart, etc.

Date and time :

Duration of teaching : 30 min

Venue :

Name of the supervisor : Teacher

Previous knowledge of the group : Identify the previous knowledge and level of understanding of patient of group

General Objectives

_____

_____

_____

_____

_____

Specific Objectives

_____

_____

_____

_____

_____

Sl. No.	Time	Objectives	Content	Teacher/learner activities	AV Aids	Evaluation
	Time allot for each content of the topic covered	What are the expected outcomes or expected changes as per specific objectives	Introduction Topic: Definition of the subject covered. Details of the content covering causes, preventive measures to be adopted services availability	This may include different teaching learning methods to be adopted as per the learning objectives and level of knowledge of the learners	This may include the different AV aids used to make the health education effective	Questions to evaluate your programme effectiveness or return demonstration

Summary and Conclusion

Any activities or recommendations.

_____

_____

_____

_____

_____

References

_____

_____

_____

_____

Reader's Notes

Reader's Notes

Reader's Notes

Reader's Notes